The Model-Actor's Dictionary

The Model-Actor's Dictionary

by

James A. Conrad

RIVERCROSS PUBLISHING, INC. NEW YORK

Copyright © 1985, 1988 by James A. Conrad

Library of Congress Cataloging-in-Publication Data

Conrad, James A., 1955-
  The model-actor's dictionary.

  1. Acting--Dictionaries.   2. Modeling--Dictionarie
I. Title.
PN2061.C66 1988   792'.028'03   88-60886
ISBN 0-944957-00-5

All rights reserved. Printed in the United States of America. No part of this book may be used or reproduced in any manner whatsoever without written permission except in the case of brief quotations embodied in critical articles and reviews. For information address RIVERCROSS PUBLISHING, INC., 127 East 59th Street, New York, NY 10022

Dictionary Guide

Cross-references are set in *italics* and are intended to direct the reader to additional information on the subject.

The Model-Actor's Dictionary

A

about-face. The act of turning one's entire body around halfway to face in the opposite direction. Also called a half turn.

Academy Players Directory. A multivolume publication listing alphabetically and by character grouping a large sampling of adult and child male and female union actors who are available for motion picture and television work. Each listing is inserted for a fee and consists of one small full-face photo accompanied by agent, manager, or answering service information. Models who are also actors may be listed here. Published several times a year by the Academy of Motion Picture Arts and Sciences in Beverly Hills, California.

accent. 1. a particular way of pronouncing word syllables that is associated with a population or region. See also *voice/speech lessons*. 2. an emphasis or distinction in style. 3. to emphasize, accentuate, give distinction to, or highlight.

accessorizing. The process or skill of matching clothing accessories to a particular outfit and person in order to achieve a correct or desired fashion appearance. Applies to everyday wear as well as high fashion.

accessory. 1. an article or implement of clothing or decoration that adds attractiveness, distinction, or completeness to an outfit. 2. an accompanying or supplementary tool, instrument, device, or container; e.g., a makeup accessory.

accessory change. The substitution, addition, or subtraction of one or more clothing accessories on a model in the dressing room or area during a break in a live fashion showing or photo session.

account executive. An individual responsible for representing clients' accounts at an advertising agency. Duties may include the promoting of agency services to clients, representing a client's needs within the agency, preparing budgeting and scheduling information, participating in the creative processes, and attending shoots and casting sessions.

accounting department. The division or section of a model or talent

10   *acting class*

agency responsible for managing the agency's financial records, as client billings, commission deductions, and relaying payment to models or talent. See also *model's account*.

acting class. Instruction in television, commercial, motion picture, video, or theatre acting that a model or actor may receive regularly, usually on selected afternoons, weeknights, or weekends.

action. 1. all that takes place in a filmed, videotaped, or live shot or scene according to the script and the director's directions or under the director's supervision. 2. a spoken instruction given by the director as a cue to begin the performance within a shot or scene; e.g., "Action [spoken softly]" or "Action! [spoken loudly]"

action photo. A photograph featuring an image of frozen action.

action photographer. A photographer hired for or specializing in shooting action photographs.

actor. 1. an individual who portrays, by way of body and/or voice, a serious, comedic, fantasy, musical, or advertising character in a film, television program, commercial, video, play, or the like. Actor can mean either male or female. If it is necessary to differentiate between the two, however, actor refers to the male and actress the female. Also called a player, role player, stage player, portrayer, thespian, or trouper. 2. an animal actor.

actor-model. Occupational title. See *hyphenate*.

actor-model-author. Occupational title.

actor-model-photographer. Occupational title.

actor-photographer. Occupational title.

actor-supermodel. Occupational title. Media use.

ACTRA. Association of Canadian Television and Radio Artists. In Canada, one of the unions for performers working in television and radio.

actress. A female who portrays, by way of body and/or voice, a serious, comedic, fantasy, musical, or advertising character.

actress-model. Occupational title.

actress-model-author. Occupational title.

actress-model-photographer. Occupational title.

actress-photographer. Occupational title.

actress-supermodel. Occupational title. Media use.

ad. Short for advertisement or advertising.

ad agency. Short for advertising agency.

ad campaign. An organized series of advertising activities designed to promote a product, person, place, event, service, company, or store.

ad layout. A plan or sketch, including copy, of a proposed advertisement.

ad-lib. 1. to perform without preparation, improvising words and possibly action. See also *improv, wing it.* 2. ad lib. One such remark.
ad sketch. A preliminary drawing of an ad.
advertisement. 1. a picture, series of images, description, or announcement of obtainable goods or services. Abbreviated as ad, adv., or advert. 2. a printed or spoken notice of information.
advertiser. The business or person doing or featured in advertising and responsible for its cost and content.
advertising actor. One who acts for purposes of advertising.
advertising agency. A company or organization representing and servicing the advertising needs of print, television, radio, film, and live promotion clients.
advertising agent. A representing member of an advertising agency or the agency itself.
advertising budget. The amount of money allotted for planning and conducting an advertising activity or campaign.
advertising community. The occupational group of persons working in or closely associated with the advertising industry. This is a general term comprising both the advertising business and social communities.
advertising director. An individual responsible for the organization and supervision of advertising.
advertising industry. The branch of business and production activities pertaining to the hiring and providing of advertising services and outlets to clients directly or through advertising agencies.
advertising insert. An advertisement printed separately and placed within the pages of a magazine, newspaper, book, mailing, or the like.
advertising model. A model who does print ads, commercials, live promotions, etc.
advertising rate. 1. the fee or charge for placing and running an advertisement. 2. the rate at which a model is paid for doing advertising work.
AFTRA. American Federation of Television and Radio Artists. In the United States, the union for performers working in live and taped television and radio commercials, live and taped television programs, and related areas.
agency. A business or organization representing and servicing the needs of others.
agency book. 1. a bound collection of headsheets, head shots, or composites of hireable agency talent. 2. a model's portfolio whose cover

has the agency's official name and/or logo displayed on it. 3. an agency's office appointment record book.

agency card. 1. a card displaying a represented model's pictures and personal statistics. 2. a small informational and promotional card on which are printed an agency's name, address, phone number, and type of business or services offered. 3. an agency policy statement card.

agency clearance. Approval by an agency of something in question, as a rate, contract, assignment, working condition, picture, or release. See also *booking clearance*.

agency computer. The electronic data-recording-and-retrieval device used by an agency to store operational information and financial records.

agency contract. 1. a written agreement between an agency and model or actor detailing each other's obligations and options by which the agency agrees for a stated length of time and percentage of the earnings to act as representation for the model or actor in obtaining work. 2. any other agreement or contract form that may be originated by an agency, as a voucher or model release.

agency director. An individual having a managerial or supervisory position within an agency.

agency division. A section or department of a model, talent, theatrical, or other-type agency responsible for the representation of a particular type of client or the performing of an in-house duty or duties.

agency inquiry call. A telephone call received at a model or talent agency inquiring about the agency's services, representation requirements, open-interview times, or the like.

agency messenger. A person or company that carries messages, business and photographic materials, parcels, and conducts general or specific types of errands on behalf of an agency.

agency party. Any party sponsored by an agency, as a dinner party, birthday party, holiday party, client party, or press party.

agency policy statement. 1. a list of instructions regarding booking and billing procedures that is given to clients. It is printed on the headsheet or separately in some other form. 2. a statement from an agency regarding its policy on accepting new clients to represent.

agency protection. Actions taken by an agency to safeguard a model's well-being. These may include the screening of clients, working conditions, photographers, and the press; also, mediating disputes and defending reputations (when in the right).

agency representative. A person employed by and officially authorized to represent an agency in possibly business dealings, public relations, talent hunts, or social functions.

agency's address and phone number. Location and telephone number of a model agency as displayed on a decal, identification tag, or card that is attached to or placed inside a model's book and tote bag. Important for returning the item if it is lost or stolen. Also appears on composites, headsheets, vouchers, talent resumes, stationery, and all other agency forms.

agency staff. The group of employees, such as one or more bookers, receptionists, secretaries, switchboard operators, or assistants who carry out the daily operations of an agency.

agency stamp. 1. a rubber or other-type stamp used to ink an agency's name, address, phone number or other information onto impressible items. 2. an adhesive stamp, sticker, or decal used similarly. 3. an agency's real or figurative stamp of approval.

agency switching. Change of representation from one agency to another for whatever reason and, if not permanent, for however long.

agent. 1. an owner or employee of a model, talent, or theatrical agency who acts as a business representative for a client from a base within that particular field. An agent obtains interviews, handles request bookings, negotiates and collects fees, deducts a standard or agreed-upon commission, and generally assists in the development of the client's career. 2. any other type of representational agent, as an advertising agent or public relations agent. 3. the agency and its operations collectively.

agent-author. Occupational title.

agent-model. Occupational title

agent-photographer. Occupational title.

agent's fee. Payment to an agent by a client for services provided. Also called a commission.

agent's signature. Found or signed in the place provided on representation contracts, agency forms, correspondence, and payment checks as a necessary business procedure.

agent's trained ear. The ability said of an agent to successfully spot voice or instrument playing potential in a person. Also called an ear for talent.

agent's trained eye. the ability said of an agent to successfully spot modeling, acting, dancing, artistic, etc., potential in a person. Also called an eye for talent.

age range. A series of ages; e.g., 18-25, graduating from young to old, any of which an actor can resemble physically in a role. Also called an age portrayal range or physical age group.

age requirement. A qualification or limitation set by an agency as part of its policy for accepting new clients to represent.

airdate log. A list containing the television stations, dates, and exact times, day and night, of when a particular television commercial will air. Also called an airing schedule, airtime schedule, or broadcast schedule.

airplay. The occurrance of airing, playing, or broadcasting on television or radio. Singular or plural usage.

airtime. 1. the scheduled time that a commercial or program will air. 2. broadcast time (hours, minutes, seconds) on television and radio that is available for purchase from a station or network directly or through an advertising agency.

album cover shot. 1. the photograph used on the front cover of a phonograph, photograph, videocasette, videodisc, compact disc, or computer disk album. 2. a camera shot whose purpose is to produce such a photograph.

album jacket shot. 1. the photograph used on the outer or inner jacket of any type of album. 2. a camera shot whose purpose is to produce such a photograph.

all-American boy. A descriptive phrase used by the print and television reporting media and in literature. Essentially, the look of a boy or young man native to the United States of America who is wholesome; upstanding in character; enjoys fitness, education, and sports; and can be likened to a role model or hero type. Also used as a casting description.

all-American girl. A descriptive phrase used by the print and television reporting media and in literature. Essentially, the look of a girl or young woman native to the United States of America who is wholesome; upstanding in character; enjoys fitness, education, and sports; and can be likened to a role model or heroine type. Also used as a casting description.

all-American look. 1. a fresh, wholesome appearance characteristic or typical of an all-American girl or boy. 2. a look, as of a product, event, or location that is wholly characteristic of the United States of America.

all-day booking. A booking that lasts an entire working day or beyond into overtime.

all media. All types of print, radio, film, television, and live communication to the public. When said of a model or talent agency, it means that they are not a specialty, or one-service, agency and will consider job offers for their clients from all legitimate areas.

alphabetical grouping. A client distribution system in a model agency in which models are categorized alphabetically by last name and then divided equally among its bookers for servicing.

alternate booking. A precautionary second booking that is arranged by a business client for the same model in case the first booking has to be canceled, as due to inclement weather.

amateur model. 1. an individual who is not employed professionally as a model or represented by an agency. Also called a nonprofessional model. 2. an unskilled model.

amateur photographer. An individual who is not employed professionally as a photographer and is without agency representation or a business base to operate from.

American cover. The front cover of an American publication; i.e., a cover from a magazine produced in the United States of America.

American look. An appearance characteristic or typical of a person, place, activity, or thing native to the United States of America.

American tearsheet. A page or sheet taken from an American magazine, newspaper, book, calendar, or the like.

angle. 1. the position of the camera and lens in relation to the subject being photographed or recorded. 2. the position of a model onstage during a fashion show or on the set during a shooting session in relation to the audience or photographer. 3. to aim or position.

animal agent. An agency or agency division specializing in the representation of performing animals for motion picture, television, commercial, video, modeling, and live performance uses.

animal model. An animal used in a photographic or live modeling activity.

animal performer. An animal used in a motion picture, television program, commercial, video, or live performance activity.

announcement. 1. spoken information by an announcer. 2. printed information as such. 3. the act of announcing.

announcer. An individual who reads the voiceover copy for radio and television commercials, program introductions and promos, station identifications, broadcast interruptions, special report notices, emergency broadcast tests, and station sign-offs. Also called an offscreen announcer, offcamera announcer, or *voiceover artist*.

annual billings total. The sum of all billings in a one-year period. This total may refer to a model, model agency, model agency division, or modeling industry.

answering service. A company offering numerous communications services, chief of which is the taking and forwarding of telephone messages to its clients. Models and actors usually have an answering service or home answering machine so that their agents and others can get in touch with them by calling one centralized phone number, thereby avoiding the problem of having to track them down. This number may be listed on talent resumes and with unions and performer directories if an agent's number is not available.

apparel. Clothing, garments, or coverings.

appearance-change fee. A fixed or negotiated fee added to a model's regular rate in order to compensate for a requested change of appearance necessary for a modeling assignment, such as dyeing or cutting of the hair.

applause. Clapping of the hands to express praise or approval. Encountered sometimes during live modeling, as at the end of a fashion show when the designer makes an appearance.

appointment book. A pocket-sized, calendar-paged book kept by a model for recording dates, times, names, and places associated with upcoming modeling appointments.

appointment calendar. A weekly or monthly calendar that is part of the model's chart. It is maintained by the agency in the booking room and is the source material for the model's own appointment book. The model obtains the booking and go-see information through a phone call or visit to the agency.

appointment record book. A calendar-paged journal used to schedule and record the daily visitors and business appointments of a model, talent, or advertising agency; photographer's studio; or hair or makeup salon. Also called an office appointment book.

arm swing. An arm movement in which one or both arms are swung in a particular manner during the course of a modeling activity. There are different arm swings for different purposes; e.g., walking, opening and closing a garment, dancing, jogging, marching, or exercising.

arriving early. Demonstration of professionalism exhibited by a model by arriving early for a modeling appointment. How early depends on whatever is standard or suggested by the model agency or client.

arriving late. A model phones ahead to the destination when running late for a booking and notifies the model agency if it has to be canceled or rescheduled, or if there are any other problems. There may be docking of pay for arriving late. In some countries, as in Europe, the policies for arriving late are more relaxed than in a market such as New York City.

arrogant look. An appearance characteristic or typical of having an unwarranted sense of importance or superiority. Also called a snobbish look, snooty look, upturned-nose look, or conceited look.

art director. An individual responsible for the design and preparation of visual concepts used in such areas as print and television advertising, magazine production, film, and video. An art director may be involved with photo layouts, ad layouts, storyboard design, and the selection and hiring of photographers and models.

artistic shot. A visually appealing and skillfully executed camera shot.

artist modeling. Field of modeling requiring models for posing live or by way of photographs for drawing, painting, sculpting, video, or computer artists.

artists' model. One who models in person or by way of photographs for artists. Also called an artist's subject.

aspiring model. An individual who desires and works toward a career, regardless of length, as a professional model.

assignment. A job, task, or obligation assigned to an individual, group, or business.

assistance modeling. Modeling done as a promotional or sales assistant, demonstrator, or handout person.

assistant director. An individual who assists a director in administrative and production duties.

assistant photographer. An individual who assists a photographer in the studio and on location in administrative duties; setting up camera shots, sets, lighting equipment, fans; and loading and unloading film.

athletic ability. 1. Being able to perform well in a physically demanding activity, as a sport, especially as applied to a modeling or acting assignment. 2. one such athletic skill or talent.

attitude. 1. the emotions or mental state expressed toward a person or activity. 2. bodily position or bearing.

attractive eyes. A physical attribute considered necessary to have in order to become a successful facial beauty model or eye parts model. See also *wide-set eyes*.

attractive legs. A physical attribute considered necessary to have in order to become a successful runway, swimsuit, stocking, lingerie, or leg parts model. See also *long legs*.

attribute. A quality or trait of a person or thing.

attribute rating. A system in which model agencies assign numbers, letters, or symbols to their models' physical attributes in order to facilitate computer or chart information recording.

audience. 1. individuals present to see and/or hear a live or recorded event or program. 2. a magazine's or newspaper's readership.

audio. Sound.

audition. 1. a tryout or reading for a part in a television show, commercial, motion picture, video, stage production, or live promotion activity before a person or group empowered to make preliminary or final casting decisions. See also *interview*. 2. to conduct or participate in an audition.

audition room. A room, office, hall, or stage where production casting sessions are held.

audition session. A session in which the auditioning of talent takes place.

audition tape. 1. a cartridge, reel, or cassette of an audition that was recorded on video or audio tape. 2. any other tape used during the auditioning process, as a *demo tape*.

author-model. Occupational title.

author-photographer. Occupational title.

auto commercial. A television, radio, or movie theatre commercial featuring one or more new or used automobiles.

autograph. The personal signature of an individual, especially of one who is famous or of noted accomplishment.

auto show modeling. Demonstrational and promotional activities requiring the services of models at new, custom, classic, and recreational automobile shows and exhibitions. Examples are as an auto manufacturer's new car spokesperson, winner's trophy presenter, and celebrity model autograph-session appearance.

availability. The state of being available for a modeling, acting, photography, or other-type assignment. Also called availableness.

B

baby file. A file kept by a children's agent who represents babies for motion picture, television, commercial, and modeling work. Each listing includes parental information, statistical data, and possibly one or more current photographs, which would have to be updated regularly.

baby model. A baby featured in a print ad or editorial photo or one participating in a live or television modeling activity.

back cover shot. 1. the photograph used on the back cover of a published, reproduced, or printed item, as a magazine, catalog, book, or record album. 2. a camera shot whose purpose is to produce such a photograph.

backdrop. 1. a sheet or structural material background used in a photographer's studio or on a theatrical stage. 2. the on-location background selected for a photo, film, or video shooting.

background. 1. the entire area behind a model or subject, especially as determined by the camera lens or as seen through the viewfinder. 2. that which is a subordinate accompaniment to the principal dialogue and action of a scene, as people, voices, movement, or lighting. 3. a person's record of education, experiences, or achievements.

background color. The single or prevailing color of a studio backdrop or location background.

background music. Music played in the background at a photo session, fashion show, fashion video, or television commercial taping or filming session. Examples of music types: ballad, ceremonial, children's, classical, country, disco, easy listening, folk, gospel, holiday, inspirational, instrumental, jazz, Latin rhythm, middle-of-the-road, movie soundtrack, new wave, popular, punk rock, rap, reggae, rhythm-and-blues, rock, soul, stage show, synthesized, techno-pop, techno-rock, television soundtrack, and vocal.

background prop. Any prop located in the background of a set or stage, as opposed to a foreground prop.

background talent. An individual or group of individuals hired to perform in the background of a production. Also known as atmosphere or, in the case of one such performer, an *extra*.

backstage. The area near and including the dressing rooms, wings, and behind the backdrop or scenery of a theatrical or fashion show stage.

backstage help. Volunteers who assist backstage during certain types of fashion shows and productions, as charity functions. Also called offstage help, volunteer stagehands, or helping hands.

back-to-school look. An appearance characteristic or typical of one or more items or activities associated with a return to some type of schooling.

backup booking. 1. a booking in which a model is hired to enhance or strengthen the presence of one or more principal models of the opposite sex. Also called a background booking or nonprincipal booking. 2. a booking in which an individual is hired and paid as an emergency substitute performer. Also called a stand-by booking.

backup child. Designation of a child on a backup booking. Also called a replacement backup child, alternate child, or stand-by child.

backup equipment. Items, such as cameras, lenses, lights, and batteries, that are kept in reserve in case a breakdown occurs with any of the primary pieces of equipment.

backup model. The designation of a model on a backup booking. Also called a secondary model, alternate model, or stand-by model.

bad side. A side or angle of a person or object considered less photogenic or visually appealing than another, as opposed to a good side.

ballroom. A large room or hall, as in a hotel, where fashion shows and other functions are held.

bare-chest shot. A photograph or camera shot in which all or a portion of a model's chest is exposed for the purpose of photographing, videotaping, or filming.

barefoot on the set. The requirement or precaution of removing one's shoes before walking onto a set containing a light-colored seamless paper or other fragile floor surface in order to prevent scuff marks or other disturbances that may show up in photographs. Also known as *footprint watch*.

base location. The center of operations and arrival/departure point for on-location photographic, film, or video assignments. Also called the principal location, base camp, or hotel base.

basement apartment. An apartment located in the basement of a building. Also called a below-street-level apartment. It is one type (although uncommon) of *New York City apartment*.

beach shot. 1. a photograph in which an ocean, sea, or lake beach appears. 2. a camera shot whose purpose is to produce such a photograph.

beautician. An individual skilled in beauty-care procedures, especially someone associated with a beauty salon or similar business.

beautiful child. An advertising character type classification.

beauty. 1. loveliness, elegance, attractiveness; pleasing to the mind and senses. 2. a physically attractive person. See also *looker*.

beauty ad. 1. an advertisement featuring a beauty-oriented product. 2. an advertisement utilizing the beauty of a model, product, location, and/or activity to sell or promote something.

beauty care. Attention given to one's body with the intent of obtaining or maintaining an appearance of healthy or cosmetic attractiveness. This is a general term under which there are many sub-headings: skin care, hair care, eye care, lip care, nail care, etc. Also spelled beauty-care or beauticare.

beauty consultant. A professional advisor in the fields of beauty care, styling, and/or products; e.g., a consumer beauty expert.

beauty contest. A local, regional, national, or international event held to select and honor a particularly beautiful and, if part of the program, talented individual. Also called a beauty pageant.

beauty editor. An individual responsible for the beauty section or department of a magazine, newspaper, or publishing house.

beauty model. A model hired for or specializing in assignments requiring significant or extraordinary physical attractiveness.

beauty print. 1. a photograph resulting from a studio or location beauty shot. 2. the media in which such photographs are found, as beauty magazines, print ads, posters, and calendars.

beauty product. a consumer or service industry product that brings out or enhances an individual's physical beauty.

beauty products show modeling. Demonstrational and promotional modeling done at general or specialized beauty products shows. Examples are as a makeup demonstrator, makeup demonstration model, hair demonstration model, or cosmetic-sample handout model.

beauty queen. A female title winner of a beauty contest or pageant. Also called a contest title holder or pageant title holder.

beauty secret. A supposedly mysterious or hidden reason, explanation, or method by which a person maintains an exceptionally beautiful appearance.

beauty shot. A photograph or camera shot featuring the beauty of a person, product, location, activity, or a combination of these.

beauty sleep. A proper or extra amount of sleep in order to maintain or promote a beautiful and healthy appearance in the awake hours.

beauty spot. 1. a small mark, patch, or mole that is real or placed on the skin to emphasize beauty and fairness. 2. a beauty-oriented commercial.

beauty symbol. 1. something that represents beauty. 2. a real or mythical person who is said to represent the higher or popular standards of male or female beauty.

beauty system. A daily or otherwise regular beauty-care routine followed by an individual. Also called a beauty regimen or beauty-care program.

beefcake model. A male model featured in a beefcake shot.

beefcake shot. A photograph or camera shot featuring a young or adult man, usually dressed revealingly, emphasizing male sex appeal. Beefcake is an expression based on the older term "cheesecake." Its use dates back to at least 1949, with current popular use resulting from media reports on male strip-tease dance shows, male beauty contests, and male posters and calendars. Beef refers to muscles, strength, and brawn. An example is a bare-chest shot. See also *hunk*.

being discovered. A moment in a person's life when talent or potential is recognized and the opportunity for advancement becomes possible. Models and actors are often asked about how, when, and if they were discovered when being questioned during print, radio, and television interviews.

bend. A modeling movement or position in which any part of the body is curved or angled while performing.

benefit fashion show. A fashion show organized and produced for charitable purposes.

best boy. One of the official titles of the first assistant to the gaffer on a motion picture or television production. Also called the electric best boy, gaffer's best boy, first assistant gaffer, or first assistant electrician.

bicoastal. Of or pertaining to living, working, or vacationing regularly on two separate coasts of a nation, continent, island, or peninsular.

Big Apple, the. A nickname for New York City, symbolized popularly by, but not derived from, a big red apple. It is a term used originally by early 1900s jazz musicians in New Orleans as a nickname for any large city or town. There was also a dance in the mid 1930s with plenty of action in it called "the Big Apple." It was first used as a nickname for New York City in the 1960s. The lighted sphere which descends in Times Square on New Year's Eve was changed to the shape of a big red apple in 1981. New York City is also called the Big Town, Gotham, Metropolitan City, Empire City, Fun City, the City of Towers, the City That Never Sleeps, Greatest City in the World, and Madhattan.

bilingual model. A model who is able to speak two languages with nearly equal proficiency. See also *multilingual model*.

billboard. 1. a board or metal structure attached to a wall or held in place by ground supports on which a large advertisement is displayed. 2. the advertisement itself. 3. a sponsor-identification program opening or closing screen title, logo, or message.

billboard model. A model appearing in a billboard advertisement.

billboard shot. 1. a photograph that is meant for eventual enlargement processing for billboard use. 2. a camera shot whose purpose is to produce such a photograph.

billing. 1. the process of obtaining payment from a business client through the presentation of a written statement, or bill, for goods or services provided, as for modeling or advertising services. 2. the listing or positioning of participants' names on a theatre marquee, movie poster, TV screen, or the like.

billing finance charge. A fee, usually monthly, computed by a stated percentage and applied to unpaid client billings.

bio. Short for biography or biographical. An account of a person's life, usually including only the important or noteworthy points, prepared for public relations or news media purposes.

black-and-white shot. 1. a photograph produced in black-and-white tones, as opposed to color. 2. a camera shot whose purpose is to produce such a photograph.

black-tie fashion show. A fashion show in which guests are requested to wear some type of semiformal wear, as a black bow tie with tuxedo or dinner jacket for men and a gown or appropriate dinner dress for women. Black tie is semiformal wear and white tie (with tailcoat) is full formal wear. Both are in the general category of formal wear.

blocking a shot. 1. the rehearsing or staging of camera, crew, and cast positions and movements before the filming or taping of a shot or scene. 2. obstructing a camera's intended line of sight.

blooper. A mistake, blunder, or error that is caught on film, videotape, or audiotape. See also *model blooper*.

blot. 1. to apply makeup, cream, or liquid in small amounts using an applicator, cloth, or sponge. 2. to dry or smooth out excess makeup, cream, or liquid; e.g., blot off perspiration from a model's face or blot one's lips (to press the lips on a piece of tissue in order to remove excess lipstick or to rub the lips together in and out slightly to blend it in).

blue-jean hibernation. An expression referring to a period of time when a fashion model is not working.

blurb. A brief promotional advertisement or description in the form of a phrase, sentence, or paragraph.

boat show modeling. Demonstrational and promotional modeling activities requiring the services of models at new and custom boat shows. Examples are as a boat manufacturer's booth assistant, boat dealer's promotional assistant, winner's trophy assistant, or winner's trophy presenter.

body chemistry. The chemical composition and processes of the human body and how they react with substances taken internally, as food, and those applied externally, as makeup, perfume, moisturizing creams, and cleansers.

body conscious. Proper awareness and understanding of one's body with regard to health or the selection of clothing and accessories.

body frame category. A classification of bone structure according to thickness. There are three categories, or sizes: small frame, medium frame, and large frame. These are the same as small-boned, medium-boned, and large- (or thick-) boned.

body shot. A photograph or camera shot that features or uses the body of a subject.

Bond girl. The media name, title, or label for an attractive actress who has had a part in one of the James Bond, secret agent movies. Usually played by an actress who has had modeling experience; i.e., a model-turned-actress.

bone structure. The arrangement and construction of bones in the body.

book. 1. a portable carrying case of soft-to-firm construction, usually zippered, handled, with inside pockets, and containing numerous clear plastic insert pages where photographs and tearsheets are stored and displayed as a showcase of one's work. Also called a portfolio. It is available in different colors, sizes, and materials. 2. to hire and schedule a model or performer for an assignment. 3. *agency book.* 4. *appointment book.* 5. *voucher book.* 6. a script book, prompt book, plot book, scene book, storyboard book, playbook, song book, or musical production book. 7. a bound work of reading, study, or business-records material. 8. a merchandise book or booklet; i.e., a catalog. 9. *union rule book.*

book cover shot. 1. the photograph used on the front cover of a book, especially a literary work. 2. a camera shot whose purpose is to produce such a photograph.

booker. A model agency staff member who takes and processes telephone inquiries and requests from business clients for models' services. Information about assignments is recorded, fees are discussed and set, and go-sees and bookings are scheduled on models' charts or computer records. This information is then passed on to the respective models.

booking. 1. an assignment, engagement, or contract to work or perform. 2. hiring and scheduling a model or performer.

booking clearance. Approval by an agency or model of a proposed booking.

booking director. An individual who manages or supervises booking operations. Also called a director of booking operations or director of bookings.

booking editor. A magazine editor responsible for assignment bookings.

booking restriction. A work category limitation set by a model. It may be in the form of a notation on the model's chart, informing the booker to exclude a certain type of assignment or category of modeling from booking consideration. Also called a booking exclusion. Examples: no nude, no underwear, no lingerie, no tobacco, and no alcohol.

booking room. A room or area at a model agency where one or more bookers operate phone lines from desks or counters, processing and coordinating the bookings, go-sees, fittings, rehearsals, auditions, and book-outs of the agency's models.

booking room call-recording system. An audio-tape recording system that may be set up in a booking room to record business calls so that information valuable to both parties can be verified at a later date. May also be operational on all lines for general security purposes. Detectable by an intermittent beep on the line, as required by law.

booking room computer. An information storage-and-retrieval desk top computer used by a booker to aid in the selection of models for assignments. Name, personal statistics, attribute ratings, union memberships, and possibly availability would be listed.

book jacket shot. 1. the photograph used on the front cover, back cover, front inside flap, or back inside flap of a book, especially a literary work. 2. a camera shot whose purpose is to produce such a photograph.

book loss. The theft or accidental misplacement of a portfolio.

book-out. To arrange a leave of absense from professional modeling activities for an hour, half day, day, week, month, etc., by notifying the agency in advance according to an established booking room procedure. Also spelled book out or bookout.

book theft. Having had one's book, or portfolio, stolen.

boom. A pole or beam, handheld or on a mobile crane or truck, on which a microphone, camera, or other device is attached and controlled.

bosomy look. An appearance emphasizing or resembling prominent breasts on a woman. An example is a cleavage look.

bottom line. 1. the final or ultimate cost, decision, or meaning of something being discussed, arranged, or negotiated. 2. a place for signing one's signature. Also called a signature line or dotted line.

bounce board. A rectangular or square board covered with a light-reflecting material. It is available in different sizes and surfaces and used by photographers to bounce natural or artificial light onto subjects or production sets in order to fill in shadows or highlight certain areas. Also spelled bounceboard. Also called a reflector board, reflector card, reflector flat, or silver card.

boutique. A retail shop or store department that sells fashionable clothes and/or accessories. See also *salon*.

boy-girl shot. A photograph or camera shot featuring a young male and female.

boy-next-door look. An appearance characteristic or typical of a boy or young man living next door who is natural looking and acting, agreeable, and friendly. He is someone advertisers believe the majority of targeted consumers would find likeable as a neighbor.

boy-next-door shot. A photograph or camera shot featuring a young model or actor with a boy-next-door look.

braless look. An appearance associated with not wearing a brassiere, or bra; e.g. a budding look or jiggling look.

bread and butter. Any type of work that provides needed income on a regular basis. For models, catalog photography and fashion shows are often referred to as bread-and-butter work.

break. 1. to discontinue or interrupt the action. 2. the pause or interruption itself. 3. a chance or opportunity. 4. to break dance.

breakdown. 1. an analysis, or breaking down, of a story, storyboard, or script of a proposed project into specific parts in order to determine production requirements. 2. a collapse, failure, or inability to continue; e.g., a shooting breakdown, equipment breakdown, or negotiation breakdown.

breakthrough ad. An advertisement of a significant nature and development in the field of advertising. Also called a first-of-its-kind ad.

breast tape. Any type of adhesive or nonadhesive tape, strap, or bandage that may be placed on or around the breasts of a female actress or model in certain theatrical or photographic situations for the purpose of holding down, flattening, covering, lifting up, or securing in place. This is done to make the individual look younger, older, less developed, more developed, nonsexier, sexier, or to help the fitting into or filling out of a particular garment or costume. Tape may also be used to hold a microphone in place during the filming or videotaping of certain scenes.

bride shot. A photograph or camera shot featuring an actual bride or model dressed as a bride. Also called a bridal shot.

Broadway (New York City). 1. a major thoroughfare in the borough of Manhattan in New York City. Times Square, City Hall, Columbia University, and the Theatre District are all located along Broadway. Its nickname, the Great White Way, comes from the past when thousands of white electrical bulbs were used to light the signs up and down the avenue. Today, lighting in a variety of colors and types is used. 2. also taken to mean the Theatre District itself, especially as the center of commercial theatre in the United States.

brochure. A thin booklet with a paper cover and pages that are stapled, glued, stitched, or folded together.

bronzer. A type of colored makeup used to give an artificial tan to the skin.

brother modeling team. Two or more brothers who work together on a regular or occasional basis as professional models.

brother-sister modeling team. One or more brothers and one or more sisters who work together on a regular or occasional basis as professional models.

brownstone. A type of building, as in New York City, constructed or fronted with a reddish brown sandstone called brownstone. It may contain offices, apartments, etc.

budget fashion. One or more fashionable garments or accessories that are in a low-to-moderate fashion price range. Also called affordable fashion or cheap chic.

building directory. A glass- or plastic-encased information signboard attached to the outside or inside wall of a building. It lists occupants by name, floor, and room number. Models are directed to clients in this way.

business. 1. a company, firm, corporation, store, shop, or establishment. 2. trade, commerce, or industry, as when a new model is taught that modeling is a business. 3. occupation or profession. 4. an actor's movements or gestures in a scene.

business manager. An individual who manages the financial and investment affairs of a high-earning performer for an agreed-upon percentage of the earnings, leaving the performer free to pursue career and personal interests. Also called a theatrical business manager, financial manager, or investment manager.

business-suit shot. A photograph or camera shot featuring a model wearing a business suit.

buyer. 1. *retail buyer*. 2. *wholesale buyer*.

buy-out. A one-time payment for rights purchased or work done. Also spelled buyout. Also called a flat-rate deal.

buzzer. A warning signal alerting all those in the immediate vicinity of a motion picture or television production set to remain quiet or proceed with caution because filming or videotaping is about to get under way. An air horn or warning light may also be used.

C

calendar model. A model hired to pose for one or more photographs that will be used on a wall or desk calendar. See also *pin-up girl*.

calendar shot. 1. a photograph used on a wall or desk calendar. 2. a camera shot whose purpose is to produce such a photograph.

California beach-girl look. An appearance characteristic or typical of an attractive, usually tanned to some extent, young girl or woman who visits the coastal beaches of Southern California frequently to sunbathe, swim, jog, or participate in games, sports, or other outdoor beach or beach area activities.

California look. An appearance characteristic or typical of the people, places, or lifestyles found in California, a state which borders the Pacific Ocean on the west coast of the United States.

California surfer look. A healthy, athletic appearance characteristic of a young male or female surfer (one who rides the crest of ocean waves on a surfboard) native to the coastal beaches of California. Usually light haired.

call. 1. a request or notice to a model, actor, or crew member to arrive at a particular place and time. 2. *casting call.* 3. *agency inquiry call.* 4. a model or performer *wakeup call.*

callback. 1. a request or notice from an advertiser, production company, etc., to a model or performer to return for another interview or audition relating to the same part. A callback indicates that the selection process is narrowing down and that the model, actor, dancer, etc., is one of a small group being considered seriously for the role. Also spelled call-back or call back. 2. a request to return for additional work on the same production, as to do more filming or dub over lines.

calling in. The practice of telephoning one's agency or answering service at a set or general time of the day or week to obtain upcoming appointments or to relay information. Also called checking in. See also *phone messages*.

call sheet. A sheet of paper listing the actors, crews, locations, and call times involved with a single day of work on a production.

cameo part. A brief, oncamera part played by a prominent actor or celebrity. It may be a speaking or silent part.

camera. A boxlike device, usually with electronic features, used by photographers, cinematographers, and videographers for taking photographs or recording images for playback or transmission.

camera animal. An expression referring to a model having sensuous qualities that can be brought out beautifully or excitingly by the camera. Also called a camera kitten, camera cat, camera tiger, or camera tigress.

camera lens. The optical portion of a camera attached to the front of its housing. It is constructed of curved or planed transparent glass surfaces through which an image passes to be photographed or recorded.

camera operator. The individual responsible for actual camera operation, setups, film or video, etc., on a motion picture or television production. Also called the second cameraman. The first cameraman is called the director of photography.

camera poise. Graceful balance, dignity, and self-confidence exhibited by a model while standing or positioned in front of a camera.

camera presence. An individual's exhibited use of body movements, eye contact mannerisms, and facial expressions in presenting an appearance and personality in front of a camera. Camera presence is the subject's reaction to an active camera and *screen presence* shows how this looks in the finished product. Camera presence may also be used to describe a model's appearance in a still photograph.

camera-ready face. A subjects's face that has had makeup applied and is ready for still photographing, filming, or videotaping.

camera's eye. 1. the round, clear glass lens of a camera. 2. the view of what can be photographed or recorded through this lens.

camera shot. A particular way of setting up and using a still, motion picture, or video camera to photograph or record a subject or scene.

Canadian cover. The front cover of a Canadian publication.

canceled booking. A modeling assignment that has been called off.

canceling a booking. A procedure established and followed through by a business client, model agency, etc., for canceling a model's work assignment.

cancellation fee. A penalty fee, usually calculated at full or half the standard rate of the model, required to be paid by a business client to a model when a confirmed booking is canceled after a specified time limit, or deadline, has expired. In some markets, a time limit is not available, as per individual agency booking policy.

candid shot. A photograph or camera shot of a subject in a position, action, or mood that was not planned or staged for the camera.

caption. A printed or superimposed description or line of dialogue underneath or above a photo, drawing, or screen image.

career scenario. An outline of a series of events one expects, plans, or would like to have happen during the course of a career.

career span. The length of time in years of a professional career from start to finish.

carpeted runway. A modeling runway or ramp that has a carpeted surface.

carpet runway. A lengthy strip of thin carpeting that forms an informal modeling runway on the floor of a room or hall.

cast. 1. to select and assign performers for a production. 2. collectively, the group of individuals performing in such a production. 3. to throw, fall, or direct upon, as to cast light on a photographic subject, cast a shadow, telecast, broadcast, or cablecast.

cast breakdown. A breakdown of a story, storyboard, or script into the individual performing parts that are to be cast.

casting agent. An owner or representing member of a casting agency. A casting agent is hired to cast all or specific parts of a production and may also be referred to as a casting director.

casting call. A notice, request, or invitation from a producer, casting agent, or casting director to submit one or more performers' photographs, composites, or demo tapes, or have the performer(s) appear in person at an interview or audition.

casting director. An individual responsible for directing the selection and hiring of actors, models, or other performers for a film, video, play, or live entertainment event.

casting office. The business location of and where casting auditions and interviews may be conducted by a casting agent or casting director.

casting session. An audition or interview held under the direction of one or more casting executive production personnel. Actors, models, or other performers are auditioned or interviewed, usually briefly and one at a time, for a particular role in a production or project. See also *emergency casting session, location casting*.

casting tape. 1. a demo, interview, or audition tape used in the casting of a part. 2. a videotape of a casting session.

catalog. A book, booklet, pamphlet, flyer, or video that lists, usually with accompanying pictures, products that are available for sale to the general public or a targeted buying group.

catalog house. 1. a company that uses catalogs regularly to advertise, promote, and sell its products. 2. a catalog production house.

catalog model. A photographic or TV model hired for or specializing in the modeling of catalog merchandise.

catalog modeling. Field of modeling in which the services of models are required by catalog clients for the photographic, video, or live modeling of catalog merchandise.

catalog photographer. A photographer on the staff at a catalog production house or one specializing in catalog photography on a free-lance basis.

catalog production house. A business with one or more photographic or video studios and other production facilities set up to produce catalogs for one or more catalog clients.

catalog shot. 1. a photograph taken for use in a catalog. 2. a camera shot whose purpose is to produce such a photograph.

catalog studio. The photographic or video studio of a catalog production house or free-lance catalog photographer or videographer.

catalog stylist. A stylist on the staff at a catalog production house or one specializing in styling catalog shootings on a free-lance basis.

catalog trip. Traveling done for an on-location catalog photo or video assignment.

catalog work. Modeling assignments in catalog photography or videography.

catch on. 1. to understand or comprehend the meaning of. 2. to become fashionable or popular.

cattle call. An open audition or interview session having a large number of in-person participants all trying out for the same part.

catwalk. 1. another name for a fashion runway; e.g., a London catwalk. 2. a narrow, suspended, service walkway.

celebrity. A famous or well-publicized individual.

celebrity endorsement spot. An endorsement commercial in which a celebrity acts as the spokesperson.

celebrity fashion. Fashionable clothing and accessories belonging to, seen on, or designed specifically for celebrities.

celebrity-fashion designer. A designer who creates fashionable garments and accessories for one or more celebrities on a regular or occasional basis. Also called a designer of celebrity fashion, designer to the stars, or a star's personal designer.

celebrity-fashion show. A fashion show in which celebrities' past personal or professional clothing and/or accessories are exhibited or modeled. It is usually a benefit fashion show or exhibition with an auction that follows and the proceeds going to a particular charity or cause.

celebrity fashion show. One in which celebrities do the modeling in order to bring attraction and publicity to the event.

celebrity lookalike. An individual who physically resembles a well-known person. Also called a star lookalike or lookalike talent.

celebrity model. 1. a theatrical, sports, music, or other-type celebrity who performs the duties of a model, as in a print ad or television commercial. 2. a model who is also a celebrity. Also called a famous-name model.

celebrity poster. A pinup poster on which a celebrity is featured.

centerfold model. An individual featured in a photograph that will be cropped, enlarged, and processed for printing as the center, fold-out pages of a magazine.

center girl. Designation of the middle female model in a modeling activity where there are three or more models arranged together. Also called the center model or middle girl.

center runway. The middle point or section of a runway. Also called middle runway or mid-runway.

center stage. The middle point or section of a stage. Also called middle stage or midstage.

Central Park (New York City). An 840-acre public park with trees, lawns, hills, lakes, ponds, trails, bridges, playgrounds, sports fields, a bandshell, zoo, ice-skating rink, open-air theatre, and restaurant in the center of Manhattan Island, in New York City. Often used for location photo assignments and off-hour recreational activities.

change. 1. the substitution, addition, or subtraction of a garment, accessory, or entire outfit on a model in the dressing room or area during a break in a live fashion showing or photo session. 2. to make such a change. 3. to make or become different, as to change a model's makeup or hairstyle, change an actor's script line, or change a production cast member. 4. *phone pocket change.*

change schedule. A chart or sheet displaying one or more names of models and the order of each's clothing and accessory changes during the course of a fashion show or photo session.

changing area. 1. the area within a dressing room where changes are done. 2. a place, spot, or clearing, usually informal, where a model makes changes in clothing, accessories, makeup, or hairstyling.

changing room. A room used to make changes. Another name for a dressing room.

chapeau. French for "hat." Used as an information heading on models' composites when translating garment names and sizes in the English language with those in the French language.

chaperon. An adult or individual of a responsible age who accompanies an unmarried minor-aged person in public or to an event. Child models and actors may require chaperones to auditions, interviews, and bookings.

character actor. 1. an adult, young adult, or child male or female actor who has the physical and talent capabilities to portray a variety of character-type roles. 2. an actor who is of a certain character type.

character actress. A female who portrays character-type roles.

character call. A casting call to see one or a group of character-type performers.

character child. A child actor or model who is of a certain character type.

character look. An appearance characteristic or typical of a character type.

character model. 1. an adult, teenage, or child model who represents or resembles a certain character type. 2. a model who is able to portray a variety of character types.

character type. One of a group or class of individuals having similar personalities or features. Examples: airplane-pilot type, army-general type, construction-worker type, cowboy type, grandmother type, librarian type, police-officer type, priest type, rock-musician type, and scientist type.

chart. A sheet of paper or thin cardboard containing information in tables, lined or blocked spaces, or diagrams.

chaussures. French for "shoes." Used as an information heading on models' composites when translating garment names and sizes in the English language with those in the French language.

cheat. 1. to rearrange the position of a performer or prop to an angle that faces more favorably to the camera or audience. 2. to trick the viewer in an artistic manner about the contents or action within a shot, scene, or edited sequence of shots. 3. to use a shortcut, mislead, or take advantage of.

cheesecake shot. 1. a photograph in which a young or adult female appears in a revealing garment or is otherwise posed displaying cleavage or one or more legs emphasizing female sex appeal. Cheesecake is an expression with a recorded use dating back to 1939. However, it may have been in use before then. It was formed by the combining of two separate expressions, "cheese" and "cake." Photographers would commonly get their subjects to produce or hold a smile by instructing them to say "Cheese." This also served as a voice cue for the taking of the picture. "Cake" is one of many past expressions associating a food item with an attractive young woman; e.g., "cupcake." The two were combined in the popular media as an informal, light-hearted way to describe pictures of smiling, leg-exposed female celebrities on the decks of ocean liners and later in reference to World War II pin-up girl photos. Cheesecake, the food, was also the main window display of many restaurants in New York's Theatre District at the time and was considered a delicacy. See also *beefcake shot*. 2. a camera shot whose purpose is to produce such a photograph.

chemistry. 1. the reaction or performance brought about by the combining of two or more individuals in a working, living, or leisure situation. 2. the science dealing with chemical compositions and reactions, as of the human body to the intake of food or application of makeup, perfume, or other substances. See also *body chemistry*.

cheveux. French for "hair." Used as an information heading on models' composites when translating personal facts (hair color) in the English language with those in the French language.

chic. Stylish and fashionable (pronounced "sheek").

child actor. A male or female actor who is under the legal age of adulthood and by law still a minor. Also called an underage actor.

child actress. An underage, or minor-aged, female actor.

child labor laws. Government regulations and guidelines covering the employment of children. In the U.S., California is one state having specific laws pertaining to children working in the entertainment and advertising industries.

child model. A model who is under the legal age of adulthood and by law still a minor. Also called a minor-aged model.

child performer. A minor-aged actor, singer, dancer, musician, juggler, acrobat, etc. Also called a child entertainer.

children's agent. An agent, agency, or agency division specializing in the representation of child models and/or performers.

children's commercial. A commercial whose target audience is children. Unless the spot is humor or fantasy oriented (with costumed characters or animation), it will use child actors or models in prominent roles. Also called a children's spot.

children's division. A section or department of a model or talent agency responsible for the representation of children.

children's manager. An individual who manages the careers of child actors or other child performers. May be a personal manager or business manager. Also called a kids' manager.

child star. A leading or prominent child performer.

child-woman. A descriptive phrase referring to a female child who resembles a woman physically or cosmetically to a degree due to early natural developments in body features and/or the applications of facial makeup, hairstyling, and clothing.

choreographer. An individual who designs and supervises dance movements in a production. Also called a dance designer.

cinematographer. One who supervises the various usages of a motion picture film camera. Also called a director of photography.

city street map. A paper folder or booklet showing a city's street layout. Used as a location finding aid by new models, location photo teams, and the like.

city street shot. A photograph or camera shot featuring or using a city street.

clamp. 1. any of the small metal or plastic devices with closeable ends used by a stylist to hold clothes together on a model. Its purposes are to make garments fit better and to help reduce or eliminate wrinkles. A clamp has more holding power than a clip. 2. to fasten, bring together, or hold in a clamp.

clapboard. A flat, hand-operated board device with a hinged stick on top to produce a clapping noise and a front surface that can be marked to display production information. At the beginning of a shot, a crew member steps in and holds the board in front of the camera. Next, depending on the prevailing custom, the scene and take numbers, title, scene location, or just the word "Marker" is verbally stated. Immediately following this, the clapstick is brought down forcibly to create a single clapping sound. This sound will be the synchronization point when the audio, which is being recorded separately, and film portions are edited together later. The crew member steps out, the director says "Action!," and the shot begins. The production information may be chalked on, penciled on, inked on, or written on small pieces of removable tape. Also called a clapstick board, clapper board, clapper, take board, number board, board marker, marker, *slate*, production information board, or shot information board.

clapstick. A narrow strip of wood or other material hinged to the top of a clapboard. Its purpose is to create an identifying sound for the audio and visual synchronization of a film during the editing process. Also called a clapper stick, marker sticks, or the sticks.

classic look. 1. an appearance of enduring or traditional quality, excellence, refinement, or purity. 2. any traditional or usual appearance, good or bad.

clean living. Honest, respectable, law-abiding, considerate, fair, decent living, as when a new model is taught that clean living will help maintain a good public image.

clean-up. The period after a fashion show, photo session, or on-location shooting when the area that was used is cleaned up or returned to its original state.

cleavage. The area between a woman's breasts, especially as made prominent by making visible a portion of both inner sides.

cleavage shot. A photograph or camera shot featuring cleavage on a woman.

click. 1. the sound associated with the operation of a camera shutter. 2. to succeed; become a hit. 3. get along well together.

client. 1. one who hires the services of a model, as an advertising agency, fashion magazine, department store, designer, manufacturer, or production company directly or through a model agency. 2. one who pays for and receives the services of an advertising agency. 3. a model, actor, photographer, or other individual who is under an oral or written agreement to receive an agency's representation.

client list. 1. a record of an agency's regular business customers; i.e., a list of its clientele. 2. a record of models, actors, or other performers currently being represented by a model or talent agency. See also *stable*.

client representative. 1. an individual responsible for representing the advertising interests of a client at business meetings and on production sets. The client rep may be an employee of an ad agency or the client. 2. any other client representative, as an agent, manager, or attorney.

client's signature. Found or signed in the place provided on work vouchers, model releases, contracts, and payment checks as a necessary business procedure.

Clio Award. An award given yearly for excellence or achievement in the commercial and print advertising fields.

clip. 1. *film clip.* 2. *video clip.* 3. a device for gripping and fastening tightly. See also *clamp*. 4. a decorative accessory containing this. 5. to cut or trim.

closed-circuit television. A system in which the TV signal is transmitted over cable and received only by one or more connected viewing sets. Subscriber cable TV is an example on a wide scale. A video audition may use a closed-circuit television monitor to view an audition in progress. A videocassette recorder-playback machine and its connected television set is another example. These are used by advertising agencies to play audition tapes, new commercials, and the like.

closed set. A production set closed to everyone except necessary members of the cast, crew, and those with special permission to be there.

close-up shot. A photograph or camera shot taken at very close range. Abbreviated as CU.

clothing giant. A large or major clothing manufacturing company.

clothing line. A variety of related garments available from a designer or manufacturer. A clothing line may be a collection in itself or part of a larger collection containing many lines.

clothing manufacturer. A company engaged in the business of manufacturing clothing articles.

clothing sample. A single representative of a particular type of clothing item. Also called a manufacturer's sample or designer sample.

cold reading. The reciting of dialogue from a script with little or no preparation.

collection. The clothing, accessories, beauty and home products, etc., available from a designer or manufacturer during a single season or entire year. The term may refer to one product line or many, as in the case of a collection made up of many lines.

color feature. 1. a prominent magazine story or report accompanied by color pictures or artwork. 2. a color motion picture. 3. something prominent, in color.

coloring. 1. an appearance of color. 2. applying a cosmetic coloring agent to the skin or hair. 3. a descriptive category or type classification used to match a model or actor with a client's needs. See also *complexion*.

color shot. 1. a photograph produced in color tones, as opposed to black and white. 2. a camera shot whose purpose is to produce such a photograph.

commemorative look. An appearance characteristic or typical of items and activities associated with the remembrance, observance, or celebration of a special event, person, or date.

commentary. A series of spoken comments and explanations by a commentator.

commentary card. A card with planned commentary handwritten or typed on it. It is handheld or kept on a lectern or desk in front of the commentator.

commentator. An individual who describes the proceedings of a fashion show or event, adding planned or spontaneous comments along the way. See also *narrator*.

commercial. 1. a filmed, videotaped, or audiotaped advertisement. Also called a spot. 2. being marketable, salable, or directed toward making a profit.

commercial actor. 1. a male or female who performs in commercials. 2. an actor who is available for paying acting assignments. Another name for a professional actor.

commercial actress. 1. an actress who performs in commercials. 2. an actress who is available for paying acting assignments. Another name for a professional actress.

commercial agent. An agent, agency, or agency division representing performers who work in television, radio, and movie theatre commercials. Also called a commercials agent.

commercial artist. An individual who creates drawings and graphic designs for advertisements, magazines, newspapers, books, catalogs, product packages, posters, business reports, promotional and sales materials, and the like.

commercial artists' model. One who models in person or by way of photographs for commercial artists.

commercial breakdown. A cast, crew, location, materials, and/or cost analysis of a proposed television, radio, or movie theatre commercial.

commercial career. An individual's knowledge and record of work and accomplishments in any of the commercial performing or production fields.

commercial casting call. A casting call to see performers for the one or more parts that need to be cast for a planned commercial.

commercial center. 1. a facility, city, or region high in the production of television, radio, and/or movie theatre commercials. 2. a business, financial, or trade center.

commercial children. 1. children who appear or are heard in television, radio, or movie theatre commercials. 2. children who are marketable as talent.

commercial client. The person or company paying the costs of producing a commercial.

commercial contract. A binding agreement to produce, write, direct, film, tape, or perform in a commercial.

commercial copy. Wording for a commercial, either that which is to be superimposed on the screen or spoken.

commercial credit. An acknowledgement of having produced, worked on, or performed in a commercial.

commercial glossy. 1. a glossy photograph of a television commercial actor. It is used for casting and promotional purposes. Also called a commercial head shot. 2. any other glossy photo used in the promotion of career or business.

commercial look. 1. an appearance suitable or ideal for television or movie-theatre commercial onscreen acting work. 2. a salable, marketable appearance; i.e., a look that sells.

commercial model. 1. one who models in commercials. 2. a character model who poses for print ads. Also called a commercial print model or real-people model.

commercial modeling. 1. modeling done in a commercial as an advertising actor. 2. character photo modeling by nonmodel types.

commercial potential. 1. apparent or developable talent for appearing or doing voice work in TV, radio, or movie theatre commercials. 2. marketing, selling, or profit-making potential of a product, person, place, or event.

commercial rate. 1. a commercial performing or production work fee. 2. television, radio, or movie-theatre commercial advertising time cost.

commercial script. One or more sheets of paper or cue card containing the dialogue and occasionally action for a television, radio, or movie theatre commercial.

commercial session. 1. a session in which a TV, radio, or movie theatre commercial is filmed, videotaped, or audiotaped. 2. a casting session for a commercial.

commercial type. 1. of a kind suitable for commercial acting or voice-over work. 2. a class of commercials, as TV, radio, or movie theatre. 3. a designation of such, as local, national, etc.

commission. A percentage of a model's, actor's, photographer's, etc., earnings paid to an agent or manager for representational or managerial services provided. Commission amounts vary among agents and managers, usually somewhere between ten and twenty-five percent. Agents also receive income from service fees paid by business clients. Also called an agent's fee or cut.

COMML #. Abbreviation for Commercial Number, an identifying number assigned to a commercial. May be found as an information heading on storyboards, scripts, and production records.

communications show modeling. Assignments in which the services of models are required for promotional and demonstrational work at shows and exhibitions featuring electronic communications products.

commuting model. 1. a model living outside of a city where modeling activities occur on a regular basis. Regular traveling into the city is necessary in order to pursue an active modeling career. See also *New York City suburb*. 2. a model who commutes internationally on a regular basis to major modeling centers to work. Also called an international model.

comp. 1. short for composite. 2. short for comprehensive drawing, sketch, or layout. 3. short for complimentary (free) ticket or pass.

competetive product. A product of a similar nature competing for the same customers or market, as one brand of soft drink with another or two perfumes. Also called a rival product or similar category product.

competetive product ad. An advertisement featuring a rival product.

competetive product commercial. A television, radio, or movie theatre commercial featuring a rival product.

complexion. The natural coloring and general appearance of the skin, especially the face. Also called skin tone. Examples of complexion types: clear, dark, fair, freckled, light, medium, olive, pale, rough, ruddy, smooth; also, "peaches and cream."

composite. A card, sheet, folder, or glossy photo on which two or more pictures of a model or actor are displayed. Name, personal statistics, garment sizes, and representation contacting information may be printed on it. Composites are used as hiring promotional pieces and are given to regular and potential clients.

composite card. A small-sized composite for models, varying around 5 ½" × 8 ½", with pictures on both sides, and possibly having foldout extensions. Also called a comp card, card composite, photo card, model's card, agency card, or Zed card.

composition. The arrangement or mixture of elements within a shot.

computer artists' model. An individual who models in person or by way of photographs for computer visual effects or animation artists. Also, one who poses for computer-generated images on viewing monitors, video recordings, or paper print-outs. Also called a computer artist's model, computer artist's subject, computer artwork model, computer graphics model, or computer animation model.

computer show modeling. Demonstrational and promotional activities requiring the services of models at shows and exhibitions featuring computer products.

condo. Short for condominum. A type of small-to-spacious, modest-to-luxurious apartment contained in a building or complex of such units. Each condominium unit is individually owned and occupied or rented out by the owner. Some rental apartment buildings convert to condominium status and others are constructed originally for this purpose. A condominium is one type of *New York City apartment*.

confection. French for "construction," "ready-constructed," or "ready-made clothing." Used as an information heading on models' composites when translating garment names and sizes in the English language with those in the French language.

conference room. A large room, such as may be found at an advertising agency, used for discussion and consultation by a number of people. Often interviews and auditions are conducted there.

confirmed booking. A booking that has been verified and is set for the day, time, and place indicated, as opposed to a tentative booking. Also called a confirmed, definite booking, definite, final booking, or final.

conflict. An incompatibility or interference with another person, product, or assignment being considered or already in effect. Also called a conflict of interest. See also *product conflict*.

conflict card. A card, list, or sheet on which a model's or actor's competetive product advertisements and commercials are recorded. Also called a product exclusivity record.

conflict-free. Free of the possibility of a conflict.

consumer beauty expert. A beauty consultant specializing in the investigation and explanation of beauty products and services.

contact. 1. *contact sheet.* 2. *eye contact.* 3. a friend, aquaintance, or relative in another or the same location or occupation who can provide the opportunity for meeting others, gaining or relaying information, doing favors, or the like.

contact sheet. A print photograph, 8" × 10" or larger, on which every shot from a roll of film is printed in its original negative size and in sequence. The pictures are inspected for quality and detail, usually with the aid of a magnifying lens, or loupe. The best ones are chosen, marked for any cropping desired, and then enlarged, using the negative(s), to the desired size. Also called a proof sheet or contact proof.

contact sheet frame. A single, miniature, framed print photo on a contact sheet. It is one of many lined in rows as they appear in sequence on the film that was removed from the camera and processed. (The negative strips of film are contacted to a large sheet of photographic paper where they develop using light into a single, collective, positive print.) Also·called a contact print frame or proof sheet frame.

contract. A legally binding agreement between two or more parties.

controlled studio conditions. The professional working environment of an indoor photographic, film, video, or audio studio, as opposed to an outdoor location, where conditions such as weather, noise, and onlookers are less under the control of the photographer or director.

convention. An organized event assembling individuals together at one or several nearby or television-linked locations for a common purpose.

convention appearance. A formal or informal showing of oneself as a participant, special guest, or visitor at an industry, membership, or fan convention. Model agents, models, actors, photographers, editors, makeup artists, hairstylists, etc., may make convention appearances as hosts, speakers, honorees, or in trade demonstrations, competitions, or book promotion/autograph sessions.

convention booking. A work assignment or speaking engagement at a convention.

convention city. A large or major city having the necessary facilities for hosting a convention. These are a convention hall, eating and sleeping accommodations, and to an extent, parking facilities. Convention cities usually have or are within driving distance of an airport. Also called a convention host city.

convention exhibit booth. A partly enclosed area or compartment where goods or services are promoted. Also called a convention stall, cubicle, stand, or space.

convention hall. A large room in a hotel or convention center where conventions, trade shows, and other events are held.

convention model. A model hired for or specializing in convention modeling work, especially at trade conventions. Also called a trade show model.

convention modeling. 1. field of modeling in which demonstrational and promotional models are required to assist clients at conventions. 2. modeling in a competition, demonstration, etc., at a convention.

co-op. 1. short for cooperative. A type of apartment having an assigned number of shares of stock in the housing corporation that owns the building. The stock is purchased by an individual who then receives a proprietary lease to the apartment and become a shareholder in the corporation. The apartment is occupied by the shareholder or sublet as allowed. New York City has more co-op apartments than any other U.S. city. 2. a shared cost plan for advertising. Short for co-op ad or cooperative advertising.

copy. 1. written material to be printed, as in a magazine or newspaper, or displayed, as on a TV screen. 2. wording that is the script for a commercial, announcement, news report, or live event. 3. a reproduction, duplicate, or replica.

copy space. The area where copy is to be printed or displayed.

copywriter. An individual who writes copy, especially for advertising or public relations purposes.

cosmetic dentistry. Field of dentistry involving the use of modern dental practices to correct and improve the appearance of teeth.

cosmetician. 1. an individual who makes or sells cosmetics. 2. a professional skilled in the application of cosmetics. Also called a cosmetologist, cosmetics specialist, cosmetics consultant, cosmetics stylist, or makeup artist.

cosmetics ad. An advertisement for a cosmetic beauty product or line of such products. Also called a cosmetic ad.

cosmetics advertising contract. 1. a cosmetics company's contract with a model guaranteeing a minimum payment for modeling services over a specified period of time. 2. a contract, usually as part of an ongoing association, between an advertising agency and a cosmetics company stating that certain advertising services will be provided and costs paid.

cosmetics commercial. A television, radio, or movie theatre commercial featuring a cosmetic beauty product or line of such products. Also called a cosmetic commercial, cosmetics spot, cosmetic spot, or cosmetics TV ad.

costume. 1. a style of clothing representative of a country, sport, celebration, occupation, period in time, or fantasy. 2. such clothing as worn by an actor, model, dancer, etc., while performing onstage or in front of a camera. 3. any outfit displayed on a fashion model or store mannequin. 4. a complete set of clothes and accessories worn at one time.

costume fashion show. One that features theatrical, historical, sports, occupational, dance, or fantasy costume wear.

costume modeling. Photographic or live modeling of any type of costume.

Coty Award. An award bestowed yearly upon American fashion designers of high merit at a gala ceremony attended by the fashion world in New York City.

counter card. A printed advertising display card found on or near sales counters in stores and other places of business.

couture. 1. the work, business, and art of designing and custom-making fashionable clothes and accessories for women. 2. the clothing so designed.

couture house. The business and design establishment of a couturier or couturiere.

couture original. The first, completed version of a couture garment or accessory.

couturier. An individual who designs, makes, and sells fashionable garments and accessories. Also called a dressmaker, dress designer, fashion-maker, or fashion designer.

couturiere. A female couturier. Also spelled couturière.
cover. 1. a protective surface, wrapping, lid, or top page. 2. the photo, artwork, or other material used on such a cover.
cover booking. An engagement to model for a cover photo. It may be used as is or as the basis for artwork.
cover girl. A female who has appeared on at least one front cover of a magazine, book, catalog, or other printed work. Unless specified, it is understood to mean magazine cover girl. Also spelled covergirl.
cover go-see. The appointment or act of going to see a client about a possible booking for a cover shooting.
cover letter. A formal or informal letter accompanying and explaining the contents of a mailing or other material; e.g., a photo submission cover letter.
cover model. A male or female model featured on a front cover.
cover potential. Having an apparent or developable appearance for being featured on a front cover.
cover residual. An additional payment to a model for the second, third, etc., use of the same photo of the model on a front cover.
cover shot. 1. the photograph used on the cover of a magazine, book, album, calendar, packaging, or other item. Unless specified, it is understood to mean the front, or top, cover. 2. a camera shot whose purpose is to produce such a photograph.
cover story. A feature article, photo report, or short explanation within a magazine that accompanies its prime or second cover photo.
cover wall. One or more walls at a model agency where magazine covers of agency models are displayed.
creation. An originally designed garment, accessory, or other work.
creative director. An individual responsible for the creation and development of ideas, as in advertising. The duties of an ad agency creative director may include the creating of advertising concepts; selecting photographers, models, and locations; attending shooting sessions; coordinating creative activities; reviewing and approving art and copy; and developing presentations to make to clients for final approval.
credit. An acknowledgement of work done. Professional work credits may be found in, on, under, or alongside photographs, resumes, bios, magazines, newspapers, books, movie posters, theatre programs, record albums, audio tapes, film and video works, and television and radio presentations.
credits coordinator. A person who organizes, files, and verifies credits for a publication.

crop. To cut short or trim off unwanted portions.
cue. 1. a sight or sound signal to or from another to begin dialogue and/or action. 2. to give or provide a person or animal with a cue.
cue card. A large card, handheld or attached to a stand, on which wording and instructions are written for an oncamera or onstage speaker to follow, as opposed to using an electronic script projection device.
custom clothing line. An assortment of garments and accessories from a manufacturer or designer that is extra fine or made to order.
cut. 1. a spoken instruction by a film or video director to stop the camera, sound equipment, dialogue, and action of a shot or scene; e.g., "Cut!" 2. to decrease or remove entirely, as to cut the cost of or cut a performer from a production. 3. to edit or change, as to cut from one shot to another. 4. film that has gone through the editing process. 5. to record sound, as to cut a record or demo tape. 6. the sound so recorded. 7. to interrupt or enter, as to cut into network programming, cut into another actor's script line, etc. 8. the manner in which a garment is assembled or styled. 9. a share or percentage of something. Also called a commission.
cycle. 1. a payment cycle. A fixed period of time used in calculating payments to performers working in television commercials, series, and soap operas. A cycle is thirteen weeks and there are four per year. 2. *fashion cycle*.

D

dailies. Daily film takes with accompanying sound that have been selected and approved by the director for shipment, usually on a rush basis, to the appropriate film and sound labs for processing and later synchronization by an editor for next-day viewing by the director and others who wish to judge what had been shot. Also called rushes.
daily chart. A model's work chart that is maintained on a daily basis. Also called a daily worksheet or daily calendar.
daily rate. The fee at which a model is paid for an entire working day,

46 *dancing*

usually eight hours, possibly from nine a.m. to five-thirty p.m., with a half hour off for lunch. Also called a day rate, full day rate, or daily fee.

dancing. A physical performing talent involving the moving of the body and feet to the sounds and rhythm of music. Used in fashion shows, commercials, television shows, films, videos, stage productions, and various other presentations. Knowing how to dance makes a performer more versatile and marketable. Examples of dance types: acrobatic, adagio, aerobic, ballet, ballroom, break, dirty, disco, flash, folk, ice, interpretative, jazz, limbo, modern, ritual, rock-and-roll, social, soft-shoe, square, strip tease, tap, and theatrical.

dancing music. Any slow or fast-paced music conducive to dancing. Frequently used to set the mood and pace of a photo session or fashion show.

darkroom. A room used for handling and processing photographic film. It is sealed from short-wavelength light in the violet and ultraviolet parts of the spectrum.

day booking. 1. a booking in which a model is hired for an entire day, usually eight hours, and paid at a regular or negotiated daily rate. 2. a booking that takes place during daylight hours. Also called a daytime booking.

day-rate booking. A booking in which a model is hired and paid at the regular daily rate, regardless of how many hours of work are involved.

daytime booking. A modeling assignment that takes place in the morning or afternoon daylight hours, or both. Also called a day booking.

deal. 1. a business agreement, arrangement, or contract. 2. to bargain, negotiate, or come to terms.

dealer commercial. 1. a commercial produced by a national or international company for its individual sales dealers across the country. Space is left at the end of the commercial for the dealer to insert a *tag*. Also called a dealer spot. 2. a commercial produced by a local or regional dealer for its individual dealership.

dealer commercial payment scale. A union fee schedule used to calculate payments to TV commercial talent performing in dealer commercials.

demo commercial. A commercial made for demonstration purposes and not for actual broadcasting or cablecasting to the public. Performers are paid a one-time fee. Also called a demo spot, in-house commercial, or non-air commercial.

demonstrational modeling. Field of modeling in which the services of models are required hour-to-hour, day-to-day, or event-to-event for the demonstrating of industry or consumer products or services to individuals, small groups, or large audiences.

demonstrator model. A model hired for or specializing in the demonstrating of products or services at trade shows, conventions, retail stores, or other public or business attended events and locations. Also called a demonstrator, product demonstrator, service demonstrator, or demonstrational model.

demo reel. A spool of audiotape or motion picture film made or compiled for demonstration or audition purposes.

demo tape. An audio or video cartridge, cassette, or reel tape-recording made for or compiled of past or current work for demonstration or audition purposes. Also called an audition tape or casting tape.

department store fashion show. One that is held in or sponsored by a department store.

department store model. A model hired for or specializing in modeling in or on behalf of a department store.

department store modeling. Field of modeling in which the services of models are required for department store modeling activities, as ready-to-wear or couture showings, or makeup demonstrations.

dermatologist. A physician specializing in the care and treatment of skin; more specifically, skin, hair, and nail diseases and the correction of surface irregularities, such as moles, brown spots, wrinkles, depressions, scars, and tatoos.

design. 1. to plan, outline, or sketch the shape or pattern of a thing or activity. 2. the plan, outline, or sketch itself. 3. the particular way a garment is assembled or worn. 4. the occupation, field, or world of designing.

designer. 1. an individual engaged in the profession of designing. Examples of designer types: advertising, animation, computer program, costume, credits, display, fashion, graphic arts, industrial, interior, jewelry, lighting, optical, packaging, production, set, sound effects, and special effects. 2. of or pertaining to a designer or designers in general.

designer collection. Clothing, accessories, or other items available from a designer during a single season or entire year.

designer house. The business and design establishment of a fashion industry designer. Also called a design house, designing house, house of (designer's name), or fashion house.

designer label. An identification tag attached to the inside or outside of a garment indicating the name or logo of the person or company that designed it. Also called a designer nametag, logo, symbol, trademark, or signature.

designer look. An appearance characteristic or typical of having been made, fashioned, drawn, or devised by a designer.

designer model. 1. a model hired for or specializing in working for a designer. This could be a full- or part-time position. Also called a designer's model or house model. 2. a form used for designing and fitting garments or accessories. Also called a designer's model form or sizing form. See also *fitting model*.

designer modeling. Field of modeling in which the services of fashion models are required by designers for hour-to-hour, day-to-day, or event-to-event presentation or fitting activities.

designer original. The first, completed version of a designed garment or accessory. It may or may not serve as the basis for one or more copies or reproduction varieties. If it does, it may also be called a designer sample and used in various promotional ways, as in fashion shows and advertisements.

designer salon. A shop or business establishment run by or featuring the work of a designer.

designer sample. A single representative of a particular type of item in a designer's new line or collection. Clothing samples are always designed in the same standard sizes and are the ones worn by models in fashion shows, fashion print advertisements, and fashion television commercials.

designer showing. An exhibition or presentation of a designer's latest collection or line of fashionable clothing, accessories, or other type products. Also called a designer show.

designer showroom. A room at a designer's business location where originals or samples of garments, accessories, or other products are on display or presented to potential retail or wholesale buyers.

designer workroom. A room at a designer's business location where designing and possibly production work are carried on. Also called a designer's workshop or design studio.

designing team. Two or more individuals associated in designing interests and activities. Examples are a relation designing team, marriage designing team, husband-wife designing team, family designing team, mother-daughter designing team, sister designing team, brother designing team, and business-arrangement designing team. Also called a design team, design group, design partners, designing partners, co-designers, designing pair, designing duo, or fashion team.

design number. An identifying number assigned to a garment or accessory for descriptive, record-keeping, or ordering purposes. An alphabetical code may also be used.

dialogue. Written, printed, or spoken conversation between two or more individuals. In a script, dialogue is construed to mean any one or more spoken lines. Also spelled dialog.

directable. Capable of being directed, especially in a theatrical or photographic sense. Refers to a person, animal, or script scene.

direction. 1. the position or path along which a person or thing is facing, pointing, or moving toward. 2. management, supervision, or creative guidance by a director. 3. instructions or orders from a director or photographer. 4. parenthetical direction. One or more instructions for an actor typed in parentheses above that actor's lines of dialogue in a script.

director. An individual who manages, supervises, and gives creative, interpretative, and administrative guidance. Examples of director types: advertising, agency, art, beauty, casting, creative, dialogue, editorial, entertainment, fashion, film, lighting, marketing, musical, photography, play, stage, technical, television, theatre, TV commercial, and video. Also called the production helmer.

director of photography. The individual in charge of motion picture photography, or cinematography, on a feature film or television production. Responsibilities include supervising the camera crew, shot composition, lens and filter selection, exposure, and lighting and film quality, all the while working with the overall director of the film. Some directors of photography may operate their own cameras. Also called the DP, first cameraman, chief cameraman, head cameraman, or cinematographer.

director's directions. Instructions, commands, orders, or suggestions spoken, written, or given visually by a film, video, or theatre director to one or more performers or crew members.

division director. An individual having a managerial or supervisory position over an agency division. Also called a division manager or division head.

docking of pay. The deducting of a portion of or an entire model's fee or wages for a penalty reason set forth in a policy, contract, or other agreed-upon condition.

dolly camera. A motion picture or television camera mounted on a wheeled platform.

double hyphenate. A person with three ongoing or achieved professions, careers, or job specialities whose occupational title, whether intended or media reported, consists of three words separated by two hyphens, as in "actress-model-author." Also spelled double-hyphenate.

doubles shot. 1. a two-shot. 2. a photograph or camera shot featuring twins or two individuals who otherwise resemble each other. Also called a twin-shot, lookalike shot, or alter-ego shot.

downgrade. To lower the status of a performer in a production to a smaller role and/or pay level.

downstage. At or toward the front of a stage.

downstage foot. The foot positioned closest to or moving downstage initially.

down time. A short or long time of inactivity on a production set.

dramatic. 1. of or pertaining to drama. 2. of or pertaining to serious or suspenseful story situations, as distinguished from pure comedic, fantasy, or musical works. 3. moving, forceful, striking, sensational, exciting, or breathtaking.

dramatic shot. 1. a photograph or camera shot featuring one or more subjects in a real or staged dramatic activity. 2. a camera shot set up and performed in a dramatic way; e.g., a dramatic-angle shot or dramatic-lighting shot.

dresser. An individual employed to assist in the dressing of another, prepare and care for clothing articles, and the like.

dressing room. 1. a changing room set up and used for dressing or costuming by models, actors, dancers, or others. 2. a room or cubicle in a retail store where a shopper is allowed to try on a garment to see how it fits and looks before purchasing it.

dressing room mirror. Any of various-sized wall mirrors found in dressing rooms. Used when applying makeup, styling hair, and checking the appearance of a fashion outfit or theatrical costume.

dressing room table. A table or counter found in a dressing room, usually attached to the wall in front of a mirror.

dress rehearsal. A practice session of a performance, presentation, or production, as of a fashion show, in which the items to be worn are used to some extent. It may be a a semi-dress rehearsal or full-dress rehearsal.

drink product advertising. Print, commercial, or live advertising featuring consumer drink products.

dubbing. The process of furnishing, adding, or replacing dialogue, music, or sound effects to a film or tape.

duplex. 1. a duplex apartment. A single apartment having an upper floor and lower floor connected by an inner stairway. Also called a two-floor apartment. It is one type of *New York City apartment*. 2.

a house or building divided into two separate living or commercial units.

duplicate book. An identical portfolio or the photos and/or tearsheets contained in it that are kept and maintained by a model or agency for various distributional or safeguarding reasons, as in the case of loss or theft.

E

ear model. A model hired to pose one or both ears, usually to advertise or promote a product or service in a print ad or television commercial. Examples are as an earring model, hearing-aid model, or ear-piercing ad model. Also called a parts model.

editorial. 1. a magazine or newspaper article, story, column, page, or photo report that expresses the ideas or opinions of its publisher, editor, or editorial department, as distinguished from the advertising portions of the publication. 2. such works collectively. 3. of or pertaining to an editorial or an assignment in editorial photography, modeling, reporting, or production work.

editorial exotic. A model having a facial appearance ideal for an exotic fashion editorial. Also called an exotic editorial model or *exotic model*.

editorial look. An appearance characteristic or typical of the models, sets, or locations used in the editorial photography field.

editorial model. A model featured in a magazine or newspaper editorial photo.

editorial nude. A type of photograph found in a magazine or newspaper in which one or more models are featured nude to some extent for editorial reasons. Also called a nude editorial photo.

editorial rate. The fee at which a model is paid for editorial, as opposed to advertising, work.

editorial request. A call from a magazine or newspaper to a model agency requesting to hire the services of a particular model so that the model can be featured in one or more editorial photos used in their publication. Also called an editorial request booking.

52   *editorial work*

editorial work. Modeling assignments in magazine or newspaper editorial photography, as opposed to those in advertising photography.

electronics show modeling. Promotional and demonstrational work requiring the services of models at shows and exhibitions featuring consumer or business electronic products.

emergency casting session. One that is held on short notice because of a sudden performer change or cast addition.

encolure. French for "neck opening." Used as an information heading on models' composites when translating garment names and sizes in the English language with those in the French language.

endorsement. An approval or sanction of a product, service, event, or cause that is acquired from or donated by a person or group of noted accomplishment, position, or fame.

endorsement ad. An advertisement using the endorsement of a person or group to sell or promote a product, service, event, or cause. Also called a testimonial ad.

endorsement commercial. A television, radio, or movie theatre commercial using the endorsement of a person or group by way of words or physical presence to sell or promote something. Also called an endorsement spot, testimonial commercial, or testimonial spot. See also *celebrity endorsement spot*.

entrance steps. Permanent or portable steps or stairs found on a modeling runway, platform, or stage.

European cover. The front cover of a European publication.

European look. An appearance characteristic or typical of a person, place, activity, or thing native to any or all of the countries of Europe.

European tearsheet. A page or sheet taken from a European magazine, newspaper, book, or the like.

European training. 1. arrangements made by a model agency to send a new model to one or more of the various modeling markets of Europe so that the model can gain experience, acceptance, refinement of the model's craft, and prestigious photographs and tearsheets for a good book. 2. any other form of training that takes place or had taken place in Europe, as formal schooling or acting instruction.

even-numbered model. A model who is assigned an even number in a fashion show production for staging or lineup purposes.

ex-actor. A former actor; a one-time or retired actor.

ex-actress. A former actress; a one-time or retired actress.

excellent hands. A descriptive phrase pertaining to a model that can be found on composites, headsheets, charts, and computer records. Sometimes coded as a symbol for lack of space. It is included for

the booker's or client's reading and indicates that the model is suitable additionally for assignments requiring close-up photography of the hands.
excellent legs. Descriptive phrase pertaining to a model. It indicates that the model is suitable additionally for leg photography assignments.
exclusive commercial contract. 1. a contract between a business client and talent stating, besides services and payment to be provided, that talent will not perform in commercials for competetive products for a specified length of time. 2. any other type of exclusive contract in the commercial advertising field, as between a business client and an advertising agency, or one between an actor and a talent agency.
exclusive contract. A contract covering a specific area of operation, responsibility, or service that will not be shared with or offered to others for as long as the contract is in effect.
exclusive cosmetics contract. A contract between a cosmetics company and model stating, besides payment and services to be provided, that the model will not do print, commercial, or live advertising for any competetive cosmetics products for a specified length of time.
exclusivity. A contract provision wherein talent agrees not to do any form of advertising for competetive products for a specified, possibly renewable, period of time.
exclusivity release. A statement informing talent of the expiration date of an exclusivity provision. If a *holding fee* is not paid, talent will upon expiration be conflict-free and able to appear or do voice work in ads for competetive products.
exercise. Many models do physical exercises alone or with a class or personal trainer routinely in order to promote good bodily health, agility, stamina, strength, and posture.
exercise on-the-go. The natural exercise a model receives while walking from go-see to go-see or booking to booking daily in a large city, such as New York City, which is oriented for pedestrian traffic, as well as automobiles.
exhibit booth. A partly enclosed area or compartment where goods or services are displayed, explained, or offered. Found in multiple units at trade shows, conventions, fairs, stores, and other public or business attended events and locations. Also called a promotion booth, sales booth, or demonstration booth.
exhibit model. 1. a model hired to maintain a presence at an exhibit booth or similar location where promotional, demonstrational, or sales activities are performed on behalf of a business client. Also

called an exhibit assistant, exhibitor's assistant, exhibit hostess, exhibit representative, sales assistant, booth model, booth hostess, booth assistant, booth representative, display assistant, promotional assistant, special assistant, information handout model, trade show model, or convention model. 2. a structural display; i.e., a display model.

exit steps. Departure steps or stairs located on a modeling runway, platform, or stage.

ex-model. A former model; a one-time or retired model.

exotic fashion editorial. A magazine or newspaper photo editorial featuring an exotic theme and using one or more exotic-looking models, fashions, locations, and/or props.

exotic look. An appearance characteristic or suggestive of being strangely beautiful, charmingly unfamiliar, or deeply foreign in nature.

exotic model. A model whose facial features chiefly suggest an exotic look. May also be called an *editorial exotic*.

exterior. Situated outside a building or other structure; outdoors. Abbreviated as EXT. or ext.

extra. An individual hired to perform a minor part in a motion picture, television program, commercial, video, or other-type production. Also called a background player, background performer, or *background talent*.

extreme editorial look. An editorial look that is very unusual, different, or extravagant.

eye candy. Something designed, added, exposed, or protruding that is visually attractive or daring, as a piece of sparkling jewelry or cleavage due to a revealing garment.

eye contact. The direction, degree, and manner in which a model fixes his or her eyesight on an object, person, audience, or camera lens; e.g., to make eye contact or look someone right in the eye.

eye model. A model hired for a photo or television assignment requiring the modeling of one or both eyes, usually to advertise a beauty or vision product or service. Also called a parts model. See also *attractive eyes*.

eye product advertising. Print, commercial, or live advertising featuring eye beauty or care products.

eye product commercial. A commercial featuring one or more eye beauty or care products. Also called an eye product spot.

F

face modeling. Assignments requiring the photographic or live modeling of the face; e.g., magazine cover modeling, portrait modeling, profile modeling, face photo modeling, face product modeling, or as a facial makeup subject.

fad look. A look characteristic of a passing fashion or craze. Also called a faddish look.

fall collection. The clothing, accessories, beauty products, etc., available from a designer or manufacturer for the fall season. Also called an autumn collection.

fall fashion show. 1. one that previews upcoming fall fashions, usually held the spring before. 2. a fashion show held in a store or other location during the fall retail selling season.

fall forecast. A prediction or look ahead as to what the fashion trends will be in the upcoming fall season.

fall line. A variety of related items, as a line of coats, available from a designer or manufacturer for the fall season.

fall look. An appearance characteristic or typical of the fall clothing or weather season.

fall season. One of the four weather periods into which a year is divided and one of the two major fashion seasons. The other is the spring season. Also called the autumn season or (for fashion) fall-winter season.

fall showing. An exhibition or presentation of a designer's or manufacturer's fashionable clothes, accessories, or other products held at a time before or during the fall season. Also called a fall show.

family-oriented ad. 1. one that is suitable and intended for viewing by the entire family. 2. an advertisement featuring a family living situation. Also called a family situation ad or family storyline ad.

famous-face model. A model whose face is well known to the public from print ads, television commercials, magazine covers, and/or paparazzi photos. Also called a celebrity model or supermodel.

famous-name model. A model whose name is well known to the public from print stories and mentions, photo captions, television news and talk show appearances, and/or acting roles. Also called a household-name model, top-name model, or celebrity model.

fan. 1. any of various electrical motor or combustion engine powered devices used to create a controlled current of air in a motion picture, television, video, or photographic studio or outdoor location. See also *wind machine*. 2. a handheld, human-powered fan used as a prop. Examples: hand fan, folding fan, palm leaf fan, feather fan, and geisha fan. 3. to move or circulate the air with a fan; e.g., power fan a model's hair. 4. a person who is an enthusiastic follower, devotee, or admirer, as of an activity or another person.

fantasy sell. The using of highly imaginative images and ideas to sell or promote something.

fashion. 1. the current standard or style in clothing, lifestyle, entertainment, etc. 2. one or more garments or accessories in the current style. 3. one or more garments or accessories of a prevailing standard or style; e.g., historical fashion, occupational fashion, ritual fashion, or futuristic fashion. 4. of or pertaining to clothing; e.g., a fashion accessory. 5. relating to, concerned with, involving, or denoting the current style. An adjective used commonly in advertising; e.g., fashion jeans or fashion sunglasses. 6. the industry, world, field, or profession in which new clothing and accessory products are designed, made, promoted, reported on, and sold. Also called fashiondom. 7. to design, style, shape, or pattern. 8. a manner or way of doing something; e.g., in such a fashion.

fashion ad. An advertisement featuring fashionable clothes and/or accessories.

fashion advertising. Field of advertising dealing with the promoting and announcing of fashion products, events, and services.

Fashion Avenue (New York City). The official dual name for Seventh Avenue in the borough of Manhattan.

fashion booking. One involving any type of fashion-related work.

fashion candy. 1. designer-inspired confections. Also called designer candy, designer sweets, or premium candy. 2. jewelry and sometimes sequins, braid, edging, trim, lace, and ribbon. Also called fashion sweeteners.

fashion center. An establishment, facility, complex, district, city, or region high in the design, production, and/or sale of new fashions.

fashion commercial. A commercial featuring fashionable clothing and/or accessory products. Also called a fashion spot or fashion ad.

fashion community. The occupational group of persons working in or closely associated with the fashion industry. This is a general term comprising both the fashion business and social communities.

fashion consultant. A professional advisor in the buying, wearing, and possibly business side of fashion. Also called a fashion advisor, fashion expert, fashion authority, fashion pro, wardrobe consultant, wardrobe advisor, or wardrobe artist.

fashion coordinator. An individual responsible for coordinating fashion shows, events, displays, merchandise, and the like.

fashion cycle. 1. a regularly recurring fashion period or season, as the fall season, spring season, or back-to-school season. 2. a regularly recurring fashion trend; i.e., fashion repeating itself, fashion renewed, being back in fashion or back in style.

fashion designer. An individual, male or female, who designs fashionable clothes and accessories. Also called a couturier (male) or couturiere (female).

fashion editor. An individual responsible for the fashion editorial department or section of a magazine or newspaper. Duties may include the planning, coordinating, and directing of editorial fashion activities; evaluating publication material and new fashions; and the selecting of models, photographers, locations, and story themes.

fashion editorial. An article, story, photo report, or the like expressing the fashion-related ideas or opinions of a magazine's or newspaper's publisher, editor, or editors.

fashion feature. A prominent magazine or newspaper article, story, or photo report on a fashion-related topic.

fashion field. 1. the realm of activities, knowledge, and interests associated with working in the fashion industry. 2. a particular category of work within the fashion industry.

fashion house. A fashion design, manufacturing, and/or sales establishment. Also called a couture house or designer house.

fashion illustration. 1. an explanatory representation, as a drawing or sketch, or even a black-and-white or color photo, of a fashionable garment or accessory. The item may be featured separately or on a model. Also called a fashion drawing or fashion sketch. 2. the world, field, or profession in which fashion illustrations are drawn and sold.

fashion illustrator. An artist hired for or specializing in the drawing of fashion illustrations for magazine and newspaper ads, catalogs, and pattern books. Also called a fashion artist, fashion drawer, or fashion sketcher.

fashion illustrators' model. A model hired for or specializing in posing

58 fashion industry

for fashion illustrations. Also called a fashion illustration model or fashion artists' model.

fashion industry. The branch of manufacturing and business activities pertaining to the design, production, and marketing of new clothing and accessory products. Also called the clothing industry, garment industry, apparel industry, fashion business, clothing business, garment business, apparel business, or rag trade.

fashion layout. An arrangement of fashion photos or drawings found in or laid out for use in a magazine or newspaper.

fashion leader. A person, company, or publication that acts as an intentional or unintentional fashion guide or exemplar for the public. Also called a fashion trend-setter or fashion pacesetter.

fashion look. An appearance characteristic or typical of the design, color, and material qualities associated with fashionable clothes and accessories.

fashion magazine. A print or television magazine whose reporting interests are the worlds of fashionable clothing, accessories, trends, events, people, beauty, health, and/or lifestyles.

fashion market. 1. an establishment or facility where fashion design, production, and/or sales activities occur on a regular basis. 2. a consumer buying group, city, region, or country where there is a demand for one or more kinds of fashion.

fashion marketing consultant. A professional advisor in fashion trends and marketing strategies. Also called a fashion marketing advisor, fashion marketing specialist, fashion marketing expert, fashion marketing pro, fashion trend expert, or fashion merchandising consultant.

fashion model. A model hired for or specializing in the live, photographic, or video modeling of fashionable clothes and accessories.

fashion modeling. Field of modeling in which the services of models are required by designers, manufacturers, department stores, magazines, catalog houses, and others for the live, photographic, or video modeling of fashionable clothes and accessories.

fashion photo. A photograph featuring one or more fashionable clothing and/or accessory products.

fashion photographer. A photographer hired for or specializing in the shooting of photographs of clothing, accessories, people, and events relating to fashion.

fashion plate. A person who consistently wears the latest fashions.

fashion pose. A bodily position taken and held while modeling fashionable garments and/or accessories.

fashion press. 1. fashion reporting magazines, newspapers, columns, and fashion broadcast and cablecast media collectively. Also called the fashion news media. 2. collectively, individuals who work in and report fashion news.

fashion press photographer. A photographer hired for or specializing in shooting photographs for reporting fashion magazines, newspapers, and the like.

fashion reporter. An individual who gathers and reports fashion news. Also called a fashion news writer, fashion writer, fashion journalist, fashion columnist, or fashion correspondent.

fashion season. Traditionally, the two biggest fashion seasons of the year are in the spring, when the upcoming fall, or autumn, collections are previewed, and in the fall, when next year's spring collections are similarly presented. Showing are held six months in advance in order to allow time for the ordering, manufacturing, and shipping of items to stores just before the start of the calendar selling season, which is actually two weather seasons combined into one, as the spring-summer season and the fall-winter season.

fashion sense. Awareness and understanding of proper fashion dressing. Also called fashion savy, a feel for fashion, a flair for fashion, fashion knowledge, fashion I.Q., or fashion know-how.

fashion show. 1. an exhibition or presentation of a designer's or manufacturer's latest collection or line of fashionable garments and/or accessories. Also called a fashion showing. 2. any other showing of fashions, as a historial costume show.

fashion show model. A model hired for or specializing in the modeling of fashionable clothing and accessories at fashion shows. Also called a runway model or ramp model.

fashion show modeling. Field of modeling in which the services of models are required by designers, manufacturers, department stores, clothing stores, magazines, and other clients for live modeling at fashion shows. Also called runway modeling.

fashion show music. Any type of *background music* used in a fashion show. Its purpose is to put the audience in the proper mood for the presentation and also acts as a movement guide for the models.

fashion show photo. A photograph featuring events happening onstage, offstage, or backstage at a fashion show.

fashion show photographer. A photographer hired for or specializing in shooting photographs of fashion show activities. Also called a runway photographer.

fashion show program 1. a plan or schedule of events and items to be presented at a fashion show. 2. a television program that reports on the events of one or more fashion shows.

fashion show see-through. A garment modeled at a fashion show that has sheer or transparent features. Also called a peekaboo.

fashion show theme. 1. a topic, idea, or trend on which a fashion show production in based. 2. fashion show theme music.

fashion show trip. Traveling done to get to an out-of-town fashion show.

fashion show video. 1. a videotaped recording of a fashion show shot by a crew from the media, designer, or manufacturer for later viewing or promotional use. 2. such works collectively. 3. the television portion of a *video-assisted fashion show*.

fashion sitting. A photo session involving the posed modeling of fashionable clothes and/or accessories.

fashion statement. A declaration, announcement, or communication, as by the use of a distinctly expressed design or outfitting technique, of a new or revived fashion idea, theme, or trend.

fashion story. 1. a media article or report pertaining to fashion. 2. fashion words, messages, and statements. 3. an idea or theme expressed visually by a model while exhibiting clothes in a fashion show. Also called a runway story, fashion skit, runway skit, or runway business. 4. the story or plot line of a fashion photograph.

fashion trend. A course or direction of fashion style, design, or usage.

fashion trunk. A sturdy box or chest used for storing and transporting fashionable garments and accessories. Also called a fashion shipping trunk, fashion chest, or wardrobe trunk.

fashion victim. Someone having worn incorrect, inappropriate, or excessive fashion and as a result has become the subject of laughter or injurious gossip. Also called a fashion laughing stock or fashion fool.

fashion video. 1. any videotaped work whose subject is the designing, manufacturing, marketing, promoting, or wearing of fashionable clothes and/or accessories. 2. such works collectively. Also called fashiom videodom or video fashion.

fashion world. The realm of activities, knowledge, and interests associated with working in the fashion industry, especially as expressed in a glamorous sense.

fast-food commercial. A television, radio, or movie theatre commercial featuring food products available from one or a chain of fast-food restaurants. Also called a fast-food spot.

father-daughter modeling team. A father and one or more daughters who work together on a regular or occasional basis as professional models. Also called a father-and-daughter modeling team.

feature. 1. a prominent part or quality. 2. a facial part. 3. a prominent story, article, or report in a magazine, newspaper, or TV program. 4. to be made or held in prominence. 5. a motion picture, usually ninety minutes in length or longer.

featured designer. In a fashion show, event, article, interview, discussion, or store clothing section, the designer who is in prominence.

fee. A cost, charge, or payment.

fee schedule. A printed list detailing costs or payments for various services or rights. Also called a rate schedule, fee chart, rate chart, or fee scale.

festival model. A model employed to participate in the opening ceremonies or day-to-day activities of a festival, fair, or celebration. Also called a fair model, festival assistant, or activities assistant.

Fifth Avenue (New York City). A major thoroughfare in the borough of Manhatten in New York City. The New York Public Library, Metropolitan Museum of Art, Rockefeller Center, Central Park, and many well-known fashionable stores are all located along Fifth Avenue. It divides the city into east and west street address numbers, is one-way, and travels downtown in a southerly direction. Also spelled 5th Avenue.

figure model. An individual who uses his or her unclothed or clothed bodily shape to model products or pose for artwork, advertisements, posters, or the like. Examples are an artists' nude figure model and a muscle-builder model.

figure shot. A photograph or camera shot featuring the shape or form of a person or object. Examples of figure shots featuring skintight clothing are a swimsuit shot, leotard-and-tights shot, tight-fitting-jeans-and-tank-top shot, and shorts-and-tank-top shot.

film. 1. a thin, flexible sheet, strip, disc, or roll of light- (or other radiation-) sensitized transparent material, as cellulose triacetate, used for recording or projecting photographic images. 2. a motion picture. 3. to photograph a motion picture. 4. the motion picture industry, world, field, or profession. All called filmdom.

film clip. A portion of a filmed work. Also called a film clipping, excerpt, piece, segment, bit, cut, cutting, or snippet.

filmstrip. A strip or roll of transparent film containing a series of still photos that are projected one at a time onto a connected or remote viewing screen. Used in promotion and education. Also called a slide film.

filter. 1. a camera-lens glass attachment or transparent sheet of other material, as cellulose acetate, used to select and control the absorption of light by film in photography. 2. to use a filter.

final booking. One that finalizes, or confirms, a tentative booking. Another name for a confirmed booking.

finale. The closing part of a performance or presentation.

fine hair. A physical characteristic, as opposed to having medium or thick hair. It refers to the thickness of the hair shaft.

first position. 1. the point or location on a set or stage where one begins a modeling, acting, or other-type activity. Also called the starting position, starting place, or first mark. 2. the location designation given to a lead model in a fashion show. 3. a bodily position assumed first.

fitter. An individual who adjusts and alters clothing articles to fit properly.

fitting. 1. a session in which garments are tried on a model or actor to determine their proper fit and look. 2. such a session for a customer in a clothing store.

fitting fee. The rate at which a model is paid for attending and participating in a fitting session.

fitting model. 1. a living model employed on a regular basis by a designer or manufacturer to try on newly designed clothing and accessory samples. Also called a *sample model*. 2. a hollow or solid structure or shape which serves this purpose. Also called a dress form, garment form, or (accessory's name) form.

flash. 1. a camera's flash unit. 2. the sight and sensation associated with the sudden operation of a flashbulb. Also called a pop. 3. to operate a flash. 4. to show suddenly and usually briefly. 5. something bright, showy, colorful, dazzling, or glittery.

flat. 1. a type of theatrical stage scenery constructed on a flat, wooden frame. 2. without variation, unalterable, as a flat rate. 3. a one-floor apartment. Also called a simplex. It is one type of *New York City apartment*.

flat-chested. Having a relatively small bustline.

flat rate. A one-time, unvarying cost of payment. There are no discounts, surcharges, residuals, or royalties. Also called a flat fee or flat payment.

flat-rate deal. A contract in which a fixed payment is made once. There are no residuals or royalties. Also called a flat-rate contract or buyout.

flat session fee. Payment for any type of session, as a television commercial or photo session, that is calculated at a flat rate.

flipper. A nickname and one of the names for a removable dental prosthetic device used on children to replace missing front teeth or cover developing ones, as for the camera. Also called a plastic partial denture or kiddie partial.

floor model. 1. an individual hired to model or promote clothes, accessories, or other products or services on the floor of a department store, convention, trade show, entertainment attraction, or the like. The model may be required to walk the floor of the location displaying garments, handing out samples, or discussing in-house services with potential customers. 2. a merchandise sample on display in a store.

floor modeling. Any modeling done inside on the floor of a location, as opposed to modeling on a stage or runway.

food commercial. A commercial featuring one or more food products. Also called a food spot or food ad.

food product advertising. Print, commercial, or live advertising featuring food products.

footlight. 1. a light positioned on the floor at the front of a stage. Also called a floor light or borderlight. 2. footlights, the plural, is also an expression meaning the stage and theatre acting as a profession.

foot model. A model hired for an assignment requiring the live, photo, or video modeling of one or both feet, usually to advertise a footwear, footcare, or ankle jewelry product in a print ad, television commercial, or live promotion activity. Examples are as a shoe model or sock model. Also called a parts model.

footprint watch. Precautionary measures taken by models and photo crew members so as not to leave foot or shoe marks on the floor portion of a seamless paper backdrop in a photographer's studio. These include the removing or covering of shoes before stepping on the paper. If the floor will not be visible in the pictures, these rules may not apply. Whatever the case, the prevailing custom of the photographer or studio is followed. Also known as *barefoot on the set*.

foot product advertising. Print, commercial, or live advertising featuring foot beauty, care, or wear products.

foot product commercial. A commercial featuring one or more foot products. Also called a foot product spot.

foreground. The entire area in front of a model or subject, especially as determined by the camera lens or as seen through the viewfinder.

foreground prop. Any prop located in the foreground of a set or stage.

foreign-use fee. Payment for the first or additional use of something in a foreign market, as a model's appearance in an ad. Also called a foreign-usage fee.

formal fashion show. One held in formal surroundings and produced

64　formal modeling

in proper form according to the highest standards of professionalism and presentation.

formal modeling. Modeling that adheres to the highest standards of professionalism and style in presentation and form. Also called high-class modeling.

frame. 1. any of the transparent image areas found on a sheet, strip, disc, or roll of developed motion picture or still camera film, or on a videotape, a single displayed screen image. 2. any photograph. 3. to select and border a shot through a camera's lens or viewfinder. 4. *body frame category.* 5. a single or sequence of timed events; e.g., a TV commercial time frame. 6. a wooden, metal, or plastic holder of a photograph, magazine cover, or artwork. 7. a setting or mounting for a jewel or other precious stone.

free-lance model. 1. a model who is free to work for a variety of clients, as opposed to one who works for a single employer. 2. a model who acts independently without any type of representation in the process of obtaining work. Also called a self-represented model.

freeze. 1. a direction from a director or photographer to stop the performing action and stay in a frozen body position; e.g., "Freeze!" 2. to stop suddenly during or seconds before performing due to nervousness or uncertainty. Also called *stage fright.*

"From the top." A director's direction meaning to begin or start over again, as the reading of dialogue in an acting scene.

full day rate. The fee at which a model is paid for a full working day, as opposed to a half day or by the hour. Also called a day rate or daily rate.

full-face photo. A photograph featuring the entire front view of the face. Also called a full-face shot or head shot.

full fashion show. One that is of full length, presentation, and uses many models, as opposed to a mini fashion show.

full fee. The normal hiring rate or charge for a service, as opposed to a half fee or negotiated fee. Also called a full rate.

full-figured division. A section or department of a model agency responsible for the representation of models who have fuller figures. Also called a larger-sized division.

full-figured model. A model hired for or specializing in the modeling of larger-sized garments and accessories, as well as for other products and services. Also called a full-figure model, fuller-figured model, larger-sized model, or large-look model.

full-length photo. A photograph in which the entire length of a subject is shown. Also called a full-length shot or head-to-toe photo.

full lips. A facial characteristic, as opposed to having medium or thin lips. Also referred to as pronounced lips or pouty lips.

full-page color shot. 1. a page-sized color photograph or picture, as in a magazine. 2. a camera shot whose purpose is to produce such a photograph.

full-talent representation. Description of an agency having numerous divisions representing individuals in various creative and performing fields. Also described as being full service or *all media*.

full-time actor. A male or female who works in the acting profession on a regular basis from day to day or job to job and relies on this employment as his or her chief source of income or interest.

full-time actress. A female full-time actor.

full-time model. A male or female who works in the modeling profession on a regular basis from day to day or booking to booking and relies on this employment as his or her chief source of income or interest, as opposed to a part-time model.

full turn. A modeling movement in which a complete, or 360°, rotation to the left or right is performed while walking or in a stationary position. Also called a complete turn, 360° turn, 360, full circle, or full spin.

funny face. 1. a comical distorting of facial features done purposely by a model or actor. Also called a comical face, silly face, clown face, joking face, twisted face, wierd face, sour face, break-the-monotony face, "Here's-what-I-really-look-like" face, grimace, or mug. 2. a makeup application of a clown face. 3. a character model or actor who is suited physically for comedic photo bookings or roles.

fur security guard. An armed, professional guard hired to protect and watch over highly valuable fur garments and accessories used during special live and television modeling activities.

G

gaffer. The chief electrician on a film production. Also called an electrical gaffer, electrician crew supervisor, lighting crew supervisor, or chief lighting technician.

game-show model. A model hired for or specializing in working as an oncamera assistant on a television game show. Also called a game-show assistant, host's assistant, prize presenter, or game operator.

garment bag. Any of various soft luggage or storage containers used to hold and protect garments and accessories.

garment center. An establishment, district, city, or region high in the design and production of new garments and accessories. In New York City, the Garment Center, or Garment District as it is also called, is located generally in the area along Seventh Avenue between 28th and 38th Streets.

general modeling work. Assignments in any of the mainstream categories, as fashion and advertising, as opposed to limited or specialty areas, as nude modeling.

girl-next-door look. An appearance characteristic or typical of a girl or young woman living next door who is natural looking and acting, agreeable, and friendly. She is someone advertisers believe the majority of targeted consumers would find likeable as a neighbor. Also called a gal-next-door look.

girl-next-door shot. A photograph or camera shot featuring a young model or actress with a girl-next-door look.

glamour product. A consumer product, as jewelry, lipstick, nail polish, or women's fine hosiery, that is suggestive of glamorous, attractive images.

glamour shot. A photograph or camera shot featuring the glamorous nature or appearance of a person, product, activity, event, or location.

glide. To move smoothly and effortlessly, as a model walking up and down a fashion show runway with his or her head and torso in a straight posture position. Demonstrated by walking as if balancing a book on top of one's head.

glossy. 1. a photograph printed on shiny paper. 2. having a shiny appearance, as opposed to a dull, or matte, finish. Same as slick.

glowing. A complimentary descriptive term that means radiating warmth and well-being, exhibiting good health and vigor, and/or beaming with excitement or pride.

golden time. An expression meaning overtime on a paying work assignment.

good side. A side or angle of a person or object considered more photogenic or visually appealing than another. Also called a best side.

good-will ambassador model. A model hired for or specializing in activities promoting and enhancing the reputation and popularity of a company or event. Also spelled goodwill ambassador model. Also called a special ambassador, special representative, hospitality hostess, promotional hostess, promotional model, or spokesperson model.

go-see. An appointment to go see or the act of going to see a particular person or business with one's portfolio, or book, in order to have it looked at and be interviewed or auditioned for a possible work assignment.

grand collection. A designer's or manufacturer's largest or most important collection of a season.

green room. One of the names for a television studio waiting room, which may not actually be green in color. Also called a guest room or backstage room.

grip. A professional laborer on a motion picture, television, or theatre production. Also called a stagehand.

group modeling. Modeling done with other models present and performing at the same time, as opposed to single-presenter modeling.

guild member. A card-carrying dues payer of a performing artists' or related union. The term guild can be found in use by work organizations representing creative individuals in the entertainment and performing arts professions, as actors, directors, scriptwriters, playwrights, and composers.

H

hairdresser. An individual who shampoos, cuts, colors, sets, and dries hair.

hairdressing time fee. Payment for time spent while having one's hair prepared for a shooting session. The model is usually booked for this time at the normal hiring rate and not at a discount.

hair model. A model hired for an assignment requiring the photo or video modeling or demonstrational use of the hair, as to advertise a product in a print ad or televsion commercial or be the subject of a hair cutting, styling, or product demonstration. Also called a hairstyle model, hair demonstration model, beard model, moustache model, or parts model.

hair product advertising. Print, commercial, or live advertising featuring hair beauty or care products.

hair product commercial. A commercial featuring one or more hair products. Also called a hair product spot.

hair salon. A service establishment where hair shampooing, cutting, coloring, styling, setting, and drying are performed. Also called a hairstyling salon, haircutting salon, hair studio, or hairstyling studio.

hairstyling convention. An organized event bringing together individuals in the hair beauty and care professions and industries for discussions, demonstrations, and styling competetions. Also called a hairstylists' convention.

hairstylist. An individual who designs and consults on hairstyles. A hairstylist is inherently a hairdresser as well and both terms are often used interchangeably. Also spelled hair stylist.

hairstylist's fee. Payment to a hairstylist for the performing of hairstyling services.

half-day rate. The fee at which a model is paid for half a working day, usually four hours. Also called a half-day fee.

half fee. Half the normal hiring rate for an assignment or service, as opposed to a full fee. Also called a half rate.

half-hour fitting. A fitting session whose time-length designation has been set at one-half hour so that an appropriate chart rate can be applied.

half-hour rate. One half the standard hourly rate. It is usually applied to such things as fittings, rehearsals, and cancellation penalties.

half turn. A modeling movement in which a one-half, or 180°, rotation to the left or right is performed while walking or in a stationary position. Also called a 180° turn, 180, half circle, half spin, or *about-face*.

hanches. French for "hips." Used as an information heading on models' composites when translating personal statistics in the English language with those in the French language.

hand model. A model hired for an assignment requiring the live, photo, or video modeling of one or both hands, usually to advertise a hand beauty or care product in a print ad, television commercial, or live promotion activity. Also called a hand parts model. See also *excellent hands*.

hand on hip. Any of the various modeling poses or movements in which one hand is placed to the side of the hip while walking or in a stationary position. Also spelled hand-on-hip. Also called a hand-on-hip pose/turn. Both hands placed on the hips is called hands-on-hips.

hand product advertising. Print, commercial, or live advertising featuring hand beauty or care products.

hand product commercial. A commercial that features one or more hand products. Also called a hand product spot.

haute couture. 1. the work, business, and art of designing and making highly fashionable clothes and accessories for women, especially on an individual basis. 2. the clothing and accessories so designed. Also called custom-made high fashion, exclusive fashion, or prestige fashion.

hauteur. French for "height." Used as an information heading on models' composites when translating personal statistics in the English language with those in the French language.

head profile photo. A photograph of the side view of the head, including the face, hair, and neck. Also called a head profile shot.

headsheet. A sheet, booklet, or brochure on which numerous small pictures, usually head shots, of an agency's models are displayed according to the agency division in which they belong. Name, height, vital clothing sizes, hair color, and eye color are usually printed below each picture. Headsheets are used to identify an agency's represented clients collectively in each division and are distributed or made available to advertising agencies, editors, casting personnel, photographers, and other regular and potential clients. They are updated regularly. Also spelled head sheet.

head shot. 1. a photograph of the head. Usually this means a frontal view of the face and includes the hair, neck, and upper shoulders. Also spelled headshot. Also called a full-face shot or resume photo. 2. a camera shot whose purpose is to produce such a photograph.

height requirement. Any of various height minimums and maximums set by a model agency and required to be met by an applicant before being accepted into their women's, men's, or children's division. Height requirements vary between the major and smaller modeling markets. It is a general rule that the major city markets prefer tall models. The smaller, regional markets may not have rigid height requirements because their client needs are different. This may also vary from country to country. (It is best to check with the agency involved in a particular market.)

height-weight chart. A standardized table listing average weights for humans according to height and frame proportions. Also called a height-to-weight chart, weight chart, or weight proportion table.

hiatus. A break or interruption, as in the filming or taping of a television series from one season to the next. Also called *down time*.

high cheekbones. A physical attribute considered necessary to have in order to become a successful, top-market photographic beauty model. Also helpful: slim cheeks.

high fashion. 1. fashion of the highest quality and design. Price and maker are also indicators. 2. of or pertaining to high fashion. 3. the world, field, or profession of designing, making, and selling high fashion. 4. a garment-size and modeling-type category designation for female models. Others are junior and misses. A model in this category typically has a slightly taller and more sophisticated appearance then a junior or misses, regardless of age, and can model high-fashion garments.

high-fashion designer. An individual who designs highly fashionable clothes and accessories.

high-fashion look. An appearance characteristic or typical of the design, color, and material qualities associated with highly fashionable clothes and accessories.

high-fashion model. A model hired for or specializing in the modeling of highly fashionable clothes and accessories.

high-fashion photographer. A photographer hired for or specializing in the photographing of clothes, accessories, people, and events relating to high fashion.

high-fashion show. An exhibition or presentation of a designer's latest collection or line of highly fashionable clothing and/or accessories. Also called a high-fashion showing.

high-priced model. A model whose hourly and daily employment rates are in a high price range. Also called a top-rate model, expensive model, or big-money model.

high-tech show modeling. Demonstrational and promotional modeling done at high-technology products and services shows, fairs, expos, and conventions. Examples of high-tech shows are electronics shows, computer shows, communications shows, and robotics shows.

"Hit your mark." A director's direction to a performer to step or land on a predetermined floor mark or spot during a performance so that camera focusing and lighting or planned movements, such as dancing or stunt work, will be correctly synchronized. Also, "Hit the mark," "Hit this/that mark," "Go to your mark," "Get on your mark," "On your mark."

holding fee. A payment, usually a session fee, to a television commercial actor to retain exclusivity on a commercial contract for one thirteen week cycle. Additional holding fees may be paid by the client as each cycle expires and new ones begin. If a holding fee is not paid, the actor will, upon expiration, be free to do advertising for competetive products.

Hollywood (United States). 1. a section of the city of Los Angeles, California, made world famous as a result of its association with the early production of motion pictures, the movie celebrities who once lived in the area, and the large "Hollywood" sign positioned in the hills overlooking the community. 2. the American film and TV industry or community as a whole, or that part of it located in Southern California.

holographic model. 1. one who poses for an advertising, promotional, demonstrational, art, or research hologram. A hologram is a three-dimensional picture recorded on a special transparent photographic film by reflected laser light. Holography is laser photography. Also called a holography model, hologram model, holographer's model, 3-D model, or holographic subject. 2. a hologram display, setup, or exhibit.

hometown. A town or city where a person resides, or especially, where one was born and/or raised. Models and actors are often asked about their hometowns when being questioned during print, radio, and television interviews.

hotel apartment. A hotel room or suite that is rented by the week or month or leased yearly or proprietarily. Not found in all hotels. It is one type of *New York City apartment*.

hot face. A descriptive phrase referring to someone's face that is currently very popular and in demand by advertisers, magazines, photographers, and the public. Also called today's face.

hot lights. Heat caused by bright studio lighting can after a while raise the air temperature on a set, causing damage to makeup and hairstyling, as well as making a thick or heavy garment or costume uncomfortable to wear and perform in.

hot look. 1. an appearance characteristic or typical of being currently very popular and sought after by clients and consumers. Also known as the "in" look. 2. said of bright, romantic, or sexy colors.

hot model. A model who is currently very popular and in demand by print and TV clients, photographers, and/or designers. Also called an in-demand model or sought-after model.

hot prop. 1. a prop that has been heated, charged with electricity, loaded, or made potentially explosive in any way. Also called a live prop. 2. a prop that is in its place and ready for use.

hot session. 1. a photo, film, video, rehearsing, casting, dancing, music, or other-type session that is very lively or productive. 2. a session in which the working conditions are less than favorable due to personal differences between two or more individuals who are present. 3. a session that takes place in a high-temperature environment.

hot set. 1. a studio or location production set that has been prepared for still photographing, filming, or videotaping and as such should not be entered or changed except by those authorized to do so. 2. a set containing a hot prop. 3. a set located in a high-temperature environment; e.g., a steam room or burning building. 4. a set that is very lively, productive, or busy. 5. a set where the working conditions are unfavorable due to on-set personal differences.

hot shop. A workshop, studio, or agency that is currently in demand by business clients.

hour booking. 1. a booking in which a model is hired for one hour and paid at a regular or negotiated hourly rate. 2. a booking that lasts one hour.

hourglass figure. A complimentary phrase said of a female having a slim or narrow waist.

hourly rate. The fee paid to a model by the hour. Also called an hour rate, per-hour rate, or hourly fee.

house designer. A designer employed by a fashion house or fashion-related manufacturing company. Also called an in-house designer, staff designer, contracted designer, or designer by arrangement.

house model. A model hired for or specializing in working for a fashion house. This could be full- or part-time work or a position booked regularly.

house modeling. 1. modeling done in or for a fashion house. 2. modeling done in the promotion of residential real estate.

hunk. An attractive, well-developed male. Comes from the phrases "hunk of beef" and "hunk of meat." Beef and meat refer to muscle tissue; hence, a man with a muscular physique.

husband-wife modeling team. A husband and wife who work separately or together on a regular or occasional basis as professional models. Also called a husband-and-wife modeling team.

hype. 1. sensationalized publicity or promotion. Also called exaggerated publicity, artificial publicity, manufactured gossip, or planned gossip. 2. to create such publicity or promotion about a person, product, event, place, service, company, or store.

hyphenate. A person with two ongoing or achieved professions, careers, or job specialties whose occupational title, whether intended or media reported, consists of two words separated by one hyphen, as in "model-actress." See also *double hyphenate, triple hyphenate*.

I

illustration. 1. a picture or similar representation in the form of a drawing, sketch, diagram, or photograph. 2. the act of illustrating or state of being illustrated. 3. the world, field, or profession in which illustrations are drawn and sold.

illustrators' model. Another name for a fashion illustrators' model or commercial artists' model. Also called an illustration model.

improv. Short for improvisation. The act of performing without preparation, improvising dialogue and action, usually within a given context. Also called an ad-libbed routine/sketch.

incorporation. The act of forming into a corporation, as a high-income model may do to herself/himself because of business and tax advantages. This is called self-incorporation. The model's corporation would be called "[model's name], Inc."

indoor fashion show. One held inside a building.

indoor location. A still photography, motion picture, or television location situated inside a building or other structure. Also called an interior location.

informal fashion show. A fashion show held in an informal setting, as a shopping center mall or community center, or on an informal basis, as without a runway and mingling among the customers and guests.

informal modeling. Modeling done in a department store, dining room, clothing store, meeting hall, or the like on an informal basis. In a store or eating room, the model circulates among the customers, possibly answering questions and assisting in taking orders for the items being modeled. See also *tearoom modeling*.

ingenue. 1. an innocent, somewhat inexperienced young woman, as opposed to someone who is crafty, sharp, or knowing. Also spelled ingénue. 2. an acting role of this type. 3. any young actress.

inner beauty. Pleasing qualities of the mind that are expressed through one's personality.

innocent look. An appearance characteristic or typical of blamelessness, inexperience, naturalness, or simplicity. Also called a vulnerable look, or wide-eyed look.

instant picture check. The taking of a test photograph of a model or set by a photographer, casting person, agent, or the like using an instant picture camera. It is done to check subject appearance, lighting, angle, and/or composition. Also called a test shot or *Polaroid*.

interior. Situated inside a building or other structure; indoors. Abbreviated as INT. or int.

international agency. A model, talent, etc., agency that has an office or business affiliation with another agency in at least one other country. Also called a worldwide agency.

international fashion community. The occupational group of persons working in or closely associated with the international fashion industry. This is a general term comprising both the international fashion business and social communities. Also called the world fashion community.

international fashion industry. World manufacturing and business activities pertaining to the design, production, and marketing of new clothes and accessories. Also called the world fashion industry or global fashion industry.

international model. A model who has worked in or is currently being represented by model agencies in at least two different countries. Also called a world-class model or *commuting model*.

international modeling community. The occupational group of persons working in or closely associated with the international modeling industry. This is a general term comprising both the international modeling business and social communities. Also called the world modeling community.

international modeling industry. World business activities pertaining to the hiring and providing of models through model agencies for advertising, promotional, and theatrical-related modeling assignments. Also called the world modeling industry, global modeling industry, or world modeling business.

interview. A meeting between a model or actor and one or more other persons to discuss a possible job or other subject. Examples of interview types: agency applicant, audition, job, and media.

interview room. a room, such as may be found at an advertising, talent, or model agency, where assignment or applicant interviews take place.

interview wardrobe. A collection or supply of clothing articles that a model or actor keeps on hand for wearing at interviews and auditions. Often an agent or casting notice will give an indication of what to wear from the description of the part being cast. Hair and makeup styling should also agree to a reasonable extent with the type of part. Also called an audition wardrobe. See also *personal wardrobe*.

J

jeans commercial. A television, radio, or movie theatre commercial featuring jeans pantswear. Also called a jeanswear commercial, jeans spot, or jeans ad.

jet set. The glamorous group of international people who travel by jet air travel to and from fashionable world locations in the pursuit of pleasurable interests. Also called world pleasure travelers or the international set. May also be part of the champagne set, beautiful people, or café society.

jewelry security guard. An armed, professional guard hired to protect and watch over highly valuable jewelry items used during special modeling and theatrical activities.

jewelry shot. A photograph or camera shot in which one or more jewelry items are featured separately or displayed on or positioned in front of a model.

junior. 1. a garment-size and modeling-type category designation for female models. Others are misses and high fashion. A model in this category typically has a younger appearance than a misses, regardless of actual age, and models junior-sized clothing. 2. the name for a particular size studio light.

K

key grip. The head grip on a film production, in charge of a crew of grips. Also called the first company grip.

key light. The greatest source of light shone on a subject or production set. It is the key for which secondary lighting, as fill-in, cross, and back, will be based. It also serves to set the style and mood of a scene.

L

large-boned. Having proportionately large-sized bones in one's skeletal structure. Same as being thick boned or large framed.
larger-sized model. Another name for a *full-figured model*.
last position. 1. the point or location on a set or stage where one ends a modeling, acting, or other-type activity. Also called the last mark or final mark. 2. the location designation assigned to the model appearing last in a fashion show. 3. a bodily position assumed last.
last shot. The final camera shot of a still photography, motion picture, or television shooting session. It may be a scheduled last shot or unscheduled due to a new idea.
lead. 1. the principal acting or performing role in a production; i.e., the starring role. 2. the person who plays such a role; i.e., the star. 3. to be first or at the front of.
lead model. The model entering and modeling first in a fashion show, either as part of a group or as an alternating presenter.
lean and chisled. A phrase used to describe an attractive male body having a well-defined muscle formation.
lean and leggy. A phrase describing an attractive female body. Same as being called lean and long legged.
leaving booking. 1. a model has the work voucher signed by the client, photographer, or an authorized representative of the client before leaving a completed assignment. A model release, which may be included on the voucher, is also signed by both parties. 2. if unforeseen circumstances result in the leaving of an assignment before completion, the model follows standard agency instructions and notifies it as soon as possible as to what has taken place.
leggy. Having legs that are long and attractive.

legitimate modeling. 1. modeling done for traditional, mainstream purposes, as to display a fashion garment or pose for an advertisement photo, as opposed to modeling in areas unacceptable or distasteful to the majority of the public, as the hard-core sex magazine field. Also called general modeling work. 2. any professional modeling work; i.e., any modeling done at a professional level.

leg model. A model hired for an assignment requiring the live, photo, or video modeling of one or both legs, usually to advertise a product in a print ad, TV commercial, or live promotion activity. Also called a parts model. See also *attractive legs, excellent legs.*

light meter. A handheld or in-camera instrument used to measure the available light on or reflected off a subject or set in order to determine the correct film exposure setting.

limo shot. A photograph or camera shot featuring or using the interior or exterior of a limousine.

line. 1. a word, phrase, or sentence of speech, as from a script for a TV commercial or program, motion picture, or stage play. For contract purposes, a script line is sometimes defined as being ten words or less. 2. a series of words, letters, numbers, and/or figures forming a straight line, as on a page or advertisement. 3. a variety of related items; e.g., a product line or clothing line. 4. the outline, contour, or defining edges of a shape. See also *silhouette.*

line reading. An oral interpretation by an actor of one or more lines from a commercial, movie, play, or other-type script. See also *script reading.*

lineup sheet. A schedule or chart indicating the names, positions, and numbers of models and garments in the order in which they will appear in a fashion show. Also called a lineup schedule, lineup chart, pictorial show schedule, change schedule, or fashion show program.

lingerie ad. An advertisement featuring one or more lingerie products. Also called a lingerie print ad, lingerie commercial, lingerie spot, undergarment ad, or underwear ad.

lingerie booking. An engagement to model one or more lingerie products live, on film or videotape, or for photographs. Various stages of undress are required. Photographs may be retouched to conceal nudity underneath, as per individual advertiser, publication, or model booking policy.

lingerie house. The business and design establishment of a lingerie designer or manufacturer.

lingerie model. A model hired to wear one or more lingerie products, as for a magazine or newspaper ad, catalog or packaging photo, or in a live fashion showing. Also called an undergarment model or underwear model.

lingerie modeling. Field of modeling in which the services of female models are required by designers, manufacturers, retail stores, and the like for the modeling of women's undergarments and nightwear. Also called undergarment modeling or underwear modeling.

lingerie rate schedule. A special model agency fee schedule that lists rates for the hiring of models to do lingerie modeling.

lingerie shot. A photograph or camera shot in which one or more lingerie products are featured separately or on a model.

lingerie showing. An exhibition or presentation of a designer's or manufacturer's latest collection or line of women's undergarments and nightwear. Also called a lingerie fashion show.

lip model. A model hired for an assignment requiring the live, photo, or video modeling of the lips, usually to advertise a lip beauty or care product in a print ad, television commercial, or live promotion activity. Also called a mouth model or parts model.

lip product advertising. Print, commercial, or live advertising featuring lip beauty or care products.

lip product commercial. A commercial featuring one or more lip beauty or care products; e.g., lipstick or lip balm. Also called a lip product spot.

lip sync. To synchronize one's lip movements with the sight or sound playback of recorded speaking or singing. Also spelled lip-sync.

lithograph. 1. a type of print made by lithography, a high quality process of printing with special inks and a specially prepared metal plate. An example is a model's lithographed color composite. Also called a litho. 2. to produce such a print by lithography.

live audition. An in-person tryout or reading for a part in a commercial, television program, movie, video, play, or live promotion activity before one or more persons empowered to make casting decisions, as opposed to being auditioned by having a submitted video or audio demo tape viewed or listened to.

live mannequin. A living model who holds a frozen body position, mimicking an inanimate store display mannequin. Also called a living mannequin, human mannequin, or still-posed model. See also *mannequin modeling*.

live model. A living, breathing person or animal that acts as a model, as opposed to a manufactured structure or shape. Also called a living model.

live modeling. Modeling before an audience, as opposed to studio photo modeling. Examples are fashion show and figure modeling.

live prop. 1. a prop that is alive. Also called a living prop. 2. a prop that is electrically charged, loaded, or potentially explosive. Also called a hot prop.

live television booking. An engagement to model on a television show that will be broadcast or cablecast live, at or near the moment of presentation, as opposed to a booking for taped television.

local spot. A television or radio commercial produced for a local advertiser and audience. Also called a local commercial.

location. A place or site for still photographing, filming, videotaping, audiotaping, or performing live. See also *on location*.

location booking. A booking to do on-location work.

location casting. The selecting and assigning of performers for a production while on location. Also called on-site casting, local casting, or remote casting.

location dressing room. A room or other area set up and used for dressing or costuming while on location.

location scouting. The searching out and obtaining permission for use of one or more suitable locations for still photography, film, or video work. National, state, provincial, and local governments may have bureaus or commissions that can assist in this task.

location shooting. The filming, taping, or taking of still photographs at a location selected for such work. Also called a location shoot.

location shot. A photograph or camera shot featuring or taken on location, as opposed to a studio shot.

location team. The group of individuals working on a location film, video, or still photographic assignment. Also called the location crew, location unit, location group, location family, remote team, remote crew, or remote unit.

location vehicle. Any of various storage, transport, shelter, or service trucks, vans, buses, motorhomes, trailers, or cars used during location work.

location work. Modeling or acting assignments that take place at a location other than at a motion picture, television, or photographic studio. It may be the actual script location or a similar one with re-created elements. Also called on-location work, on-site work, or remote work.

lodging. The practice and customs of arriving, staying, and checking out of regional, national, and international hotels, motels, and resorts that a model or actor experiences during location work. Generally, travel and lodging arrangements are made by the client and relayed to the model or actor through his and her agency. Photo teams normally travel as a group with the client paying the expenses. A hotel, resort, etc., may exchange its services for publicity.

loft. A type of apartment or commercial space having a high ceiling that is found in converted warehouse, factory, and similar-type buildings. Photographic and video studios are usually located in commercial loft space buildings. An apartment in a living/residential loft building is one type of *New York City apartment*.

loft studio. A photographic, video, design, or artist studio located in a commercial loft building.

London-based (United Kingdom). Modeling industry colleagues and activities based in the city of London, England, the capital of the United Kingdom of Great Britian and Northern Ireland.

long legs. A physical attribute considered necessary to have in order to become a successful, top-market fashion model. See also *leggy, lean and leggy, attractive legs.*

long neck. A physical attribute considered necessary to have in order to become a successful, top-market fashion or beauty model. Also called a slender neck, willowy neck, or swan neck.

look. 1. a general or particular appearance of a person, product, location, or activity. 2. an expression of the face. See also *arrogant look, innocent look, moody look, seductive look, serious look, sexy look, sophisticated look, funny face, smile.* 3. to set one's eyes on or in the direction of. See also *eye contact.*

lookalike talent. 1. an individual who resembles a well-known person physically and on that basis is hired to perform. Also called a lookalike. 2. such individuals collectively. 3. the ability or skill to perform as a lookalike.

looker. An individual having attractive physical looks. Also called a good-looker, eye-capturer, eye-filler, eye-popper, head-turner, traffic-stopper, standout, stunner, fox, beauty, or hunk.

loop. A length of film or sound tape that is spliced end to end so that it can be machine-played repetitively. In a special sound studio, an actor or voiceover artist would watch a continually replayed "looped" scene on a screen and, using a microphone and single or dual earphones, respeak or resing those words or lyrics that need to be improved or changed. This process is called looping or dubbing.

loupe. A type of pocket-sized magnifying glass used to examine such items as print photographs, photo slides, graphic artwork, and precious jewelry. It is pronounced "loop." A base magnifier may also be used for these purposes.

lunch break. The stopping of a day-long photo session or film or tape production for the eating of lunch. Depending on the location and situation, food is either provided or available off the set.

luncheon fashion show. A formal or informal fashion show during which lunch is served or made available on a buffet. Also called a luncheon and fashion show, fashion show and luncheon, tearoom fashion show, tea-and-cake fashion show, or brunch fashion show.

M

macho look. An appearance characteristic or typical of strong, virile masculinity. Also called a machismo look or manly look.

made-up look. 1. an appearance of having had facial makeup applied. 2. an appearance characteristic or typical of an intentional or unintentional overapplication of facial makeup, jewelry, and/or hairstyling. Also spelled madeup look.

Madison Avenue (New York City). 1. a well-known avenue in the borough of Manhattan in New York City along or near which many advertising and related businesses are located. It is situated between Park Avenue and Fifth Avenue. 2. also taken to mean the center of the advertising industry in the United States, its methods, and influence on society. Also called Mad Avenue.

magazine. 1. a printed, multipaged publication issued at regular intervals whose pages, depending on the magazine's format and theme, contain articles, stories, reports, advertisements, and/or illustrations. Also called a periodical. 2. a television program that reports on a variety of general or special interest topics. Also called a videomagazine. 3. a container attached to a camera that holds it raw and exposed film.

magazine cover booking. An engagement to model for a magazine cover picture.

magazine cover shot. 1. the photograph, video still, or video sequence used on the front cover or opening segment of a print or TV magazine. 2. a camera shot whose purpose is to produce such an image or series of images.

magazine story. 1. an article or photo report appearing in a print magazine of any kind. 2. such material as presented on a television news or variety magazine program

magazine trip. Traveling done for an on-location magazine photo or video assignment.

magazine work. Modeling assignments in magazine advertising or editorial photography, videography, or reporting.

mail pickup. The collecting, or picking up, of fan mail by an extremely popular model or actor at his or her agency or other representative after it has been sent there directly or forwarded from other sources. It may also be remailed directly to the model or actor. Motion picture and television unions also receive and forward mail to their members.

major agency. A model, talent, or advertising agency that is large or formost in its field. A multidivisioned agency.

major booking. A booking that is highly prestigious or for which there is substantial payment.

major celebrity. A celebrity of the highest rank, stature, or popularity. Also called a big-name celebrity, top-name celebrity, top celebrity, major star, or superstar.

makeover. 1. a beauty session in which a person's facial makeup and possibly hairstyle are redone, resulting in a noticeably improved appearance or merely a changed one, as for theatrical purposes. 2. to perform such a session. Also spelled make-over.

makeup. 1. any of various facial or body cosmetics used to beautify, color, conceal, bring prominence to, or otherwise change one's features. Also spelled make-up. 2. such products collectively. 3. to apply make-up.

makeup ad. An advertisement featuring one or more makeup products.

makeup artist. An individual skilled in the design, construction, and application of beauty, theatrical, or special effects makeup. Also called a makeup applier, makeup person, face artist, or cosmetician.

makeup artist's fee. Payment to a makeup artist for the performing of makeup artistry services.

makeup call. A model's or actor's scheduled appointment for servicing at the makeup department of a studio, theatre, or location set.

makeup class. Formal or informal instruction on the correct application of makeup. This is eventually supplemented with on-the-job experience with makeup artists and other models.

constructing, and applying beauty, theatrical, or special effects makeup. A makeup consultant is usually a makeup artist as well. Also called a makeup expert, makeup authority, or makeup pro.

makeup department. A section or department of a production house, studio, or theatre responsible for the design, construction, and application of makeup on actors, models, dancers, news people, and others who appear oncamera or onstage.

makeup mirror. Any of various-sized wall, tabletop, handbag, or pocket mirrors used when applying or removing makeup or checking one's hairstyle.

makeup salon. A service or instructional establishment where makeup is applied or its use taught. Also called a makeup studio, makeup clinic, or makeup artistry classroom.

makeup table. A table or counter attached to the wall in front of a mirror in a dressing room. It is used for the storing and placing of makeup and accessories.

makeup trick. A clever way, method, or procedure of applying or removing makeup. Also called a makeup tip, how-to, pointer, suggestion, or secret.

making the rounds. 1. the daily or weekly activities of traveling to and participating in go-sees, interviews, and auditions in order to gain professional work. Also known as pounding the pavement or legwork. 2. traveling a regular route.

male model. A young or adult male who models professionally or on an amateur basis. It is a term used to differentiate between female models, who are in the majority in the profession.

manager. An individual who, depending on the particular field, supervises, directs, or guides an administrative department, work activities, one or more careers, money matters, etc. See also *business manager, personal manager, children's manager*.

manager's fee. Payment to a manager by a client for managerial services provided. Also called a manager's percentage of client's earnings, manager's deducted share, manager's commission, or manager's cut.

Manhattan (New York City). An island and one of the five boroughs of New York City (Manhattan, Bronx, Queens, Brooklyn, and Staten Island). It is located conspicuously on the upper west side of the city's watery boundaries. Manhattan Island is also commonly referred to as New York. New York City, with its five boroughs, is also called New York, Greater New York, and the City of New York.

manicure. A beauty treatment consisting of cleaning, trimming, and polishing the fingernails. It is done by a manicurist. Such a treatment for the toenails is called a pedicure.

mannequin. 1. a hollow or solid, manufactured structure or shape resembling the bodily form, or parts thereof, of a man, woman, or child. It is used primarily for the displaying or sizing of clothing and accessories. Also spelled mannikin, manikin, or manakin. Also called a display form, sizing form, clothing dummy, lay figure, or fitting model. 2. another name for a living model.

mannequin agency. Another name for a model agency.

mannequin modeling. An unusual type of modeling in which living models hold frozen body positions, mimicking inanimate display mannequins. See *live mannequin*.

manufacturer. A company, utilizing a factory, plant, or workshop, that is engaged in the business of making consumer or industry products. A manufacturer may have its own design department or produce from the designs of its clients. Also called a manufacturing house, maker, creator, fabricator, or product producer.

manufacturer showing. An exhibition or presentation of a manufacturer's latest collection or line of consumer or industry products, as clothing, acessories, makeup, or fabrics.

manufacturer's model. 1. a living model hired for or specializing in working for a manufacturer. This could be a full- or part-time job or a position booked regularly. 2. a structure or shape which serves this purpose.

manufacturer's sample. A single representative of a particular type of product. Also called an example, specimen, or handout.

manufacturer's showroom. A room at a manufacturer's office or factory location where originals or samples of its products are on display or presented to wholesale buyers or the media.

mark. 1. the designated location on a set or stage where one begins, continues, or ends an acting, speaking, modeling, etc., activity. It is usually indicated by a small line, spot, or piece of tape drawn on or attached to the floor or ground. A position can also be set and recorded by taking a measurement from the camera to the subject using a measuring tape or string. 2. to place a mark, as a piece of tape, spot, sign, symbol, underline, or short sound blip on something by manual, mechanical, or electronic means. 3. to operate a clapboard in front of a running camera at the start of a motion picture, commercial, or television program shot or scene. Same as to *slate*.

market week. Any of various designated weeks of the year for presenting new merchandise lines to wholesale buyers.

marriage leave. The taking of a day or more off from modeling work to get married and/or go on a honeymoon vacation. Also called a marriage bookout, wedding bookout, or marriage/vacation leave.

maternity leave. The taking of an extended length of time off from modeling work during the latter stages of a pregnancy and the postpartum period afterward. Also called a maternity bookout or pregnancy leave.

matronly look. An appearance characteristic or typical of a married, divorced, or widowed older woman who has and has had children to oversee. Also called a matriarchal look.

mature look. An appearance characteristic or typical of someone who is older, experienced, responsible, or dignified; e.g., a mature older woman look or maturely dignified look.

maximum-use period. The length of time set forth in a contract for the use of something, as a principal actor's or model's appearance in a television commercial or print advertisement.

meal penalty. A union-determined payment to actors or crew members from a production company if it fails to or is late in providing some type of meal or meal break in accordance with the length of working time.

measurements. 1. sizes, dimensions, proportions, as of one's height, chest, waist, hips, legs, feet, neck, head, arms, and/or hands. Also called personal statistics. 2. camera-lens-to-subject measurements.

media. The various forms of communication to large numbers of people. Medium is singular. See also *all media, print media*.

medium-boned. Having proportionately medium-sized bones in one's skeletal structure. Same as being average boned, average framed, or medium framed.

men's division. A section or department of a model agency responsible for the representation of men. Also called a men's section, men's department, or male division.

men's residence. An apartment or rooming house run similarly to a women's residence, but for men only. Less in number than those specializing in female customers. Most such places now admit both sexes. Also called a men's hotel. A room in a men's residence is one type of *New York City apartment*.

mini fashion show. 1. one held in limited or confined surroundings and/or is of shorter length and with fewer models than a full fashion show. Also called a mini-presentation fashion show, mini-format fashion show, or single-presenter showing. 2. a fashion show featuring short-length dresses, skirts, or pants. 3. one featuring miniature fashions, as for dolls. Also called a miniature-collectables fashion show or doll fashions show.

minimum fee. The lowest payment required to hire a person or service;

e.g., a model's minimum fee or photographer's minimum fee. Also called a minimum rate or starting fee.

mirror practice. Standing in front of a mirror and practicing modeling, acting, or dancing body movements and/or facial expressions.

misses. A garment-size and modeling-type category designation for female models. Others are junior and high fashion. A model in this category typically has a slightly older and more developed appearance than a junior, regardless of actual age, and models misses-size clothing. Also called a miss or missy.

model. 1. an individual who performs as a visual or bodily subject for a photographer, designer, artist, videographer, filmmaker, or the like. Also called a poser. 2. an individual who is hired, primarily on the basis of his or her level of physical beauty or uniqueness, to perform as a displayer, presenter, demonstrator, or promoter of a product or service. Also called a mannequin. 3. an animal or object which serves in either of these capacities. Also called a subject, figure, or form. 4. a representative of something; e.g., a role model, product model, etc. 5. to pose, display, present, demonstrate, promote, or assist as a model.

model-actor. A model who also works as an actor; a model and actor. An occupational title. Pronounced "model actor" or "model hyphen actor." Other forms: model-and-actor, model/actor ("model and/or actor" or "model slash actor"). See *hyphenate*.

model-actor-author. Occupational title.

model-actor-photographer. Occupational title.

model-actress. Occupational title.

model-actress-author. Occupational title.

model-actress-photographer. Occupational title.

model agency. A representational business working on a commission basis and whose clients are models. Also called a modeling agency, mannequin agency, or fashion agency.

model agent. 1. an owner or employee of a model agency who acts as a business representative for a model from a base within the modeling industry. A model agent, alone or using a staff, obtains interviews, handles request bookings, negotiates and collects fees, deducts a standard or agreed-upon commission, and generally assists in the development of the model's career. Also called a modeling agent, models' agent, mannequin agent, model representative, models' rep, model rep, or *print agent*. 2. the agency and its operations collectively. Also called a model business, modeling business, supplier of models, or supplier of modeling talent.

model as actor. Modeling is increasingly being recognized to be a type of silent acting. A model, just as an actor, is made-up, costumed, and guided in performing by a script or the spoken directions of another individual. Both work in front of a camera or live audience. Print and TV commercial modeling are highly visible fields to producers and casting people are considered to be viable stepping stones to getting small and major parts in feature films, videos, and television movies, series, programs, and specials. Models who would like their careers to turn toward full-time acting supplement their modeling with part-time acting lessons. See also *print actor*.

model-author. Occupational title.

model blooper. A mistake, blunder, or error, especially one that is recorded visually or by sound, made or experienced by a model. Also called a modeling blooper.

model burnout. The condition of being exhausted, used up, or worn out mentally or physically as a model. Also called model fatigue.

model candidate. An individual who has the possibility of or who has chosen to seek out becoming a model. Also referred to as model material.

model chaser. A person, male or female, who actively seeks the social company of one or more beauty models primarily for reasons of physical gratification and the status-seeking desire to be seen and associated with such individuals. Should not be confused with a sincere person and relationship. Also spelled model-chaser. See also *professional model chaser*.

model-dancer. Occupational title.

model-designer. Occupational title.

model development. The process of learning how to live and work correctly and successfully as a model. Also called professional model development, model learning, model training, modeling instruction, on-the-job training, or on-the-job experience.

model face. 1. a face associated with models. Also called a model's face or model-like face. See also *hot face, new face, today's face*. 2. a person having such a face. A nickname.

modeling. 1. performing; i.e., posing, displaying, demonstrating, promoting, or assisting using body and/or facial movements, as a model. 2. the industry, world, field, or profession, in which models and others work. Also called the modeling profession, modeling business, or modeldom.

modeling bag. Any of various-sized, soft construction tote bags used by a model to hold and protect garments, accessories, makeup, hair-care items, and other personal articles while traveling to and from modeling assignments.

modeling career. An individual's knowledge and record of work and accomplishments in any or all of the various fields of modeling.

modeling center. 1. an establishment where modeling activities take place. Also called a modeling studio, modeling school, or modeling facility. 2. a city or region with a high volume of modeling activities. Also called a center of modeling or modeling capital.

modeling community. The occupational group of persons working in or closely associated with the modeling industry. This is a general term comprising both the modeling business and social communities. Also called the modeling crowd, modeling circle, modeling club, or model club.

modeling contest. 1. a local, regional, national, or international event or search operation conducted by a model agency, beauty/fashion magazine, etc., to find and award new and outstanding beauty or fashion modeling talent. Examples are a photo model contest, cover model contest, live modeling contest, modeling competition, new model search, or talent search. 2. any other event or program to select, honor, or recognize new or established models.

modeling contract. A contract for or representing a model's services.

modeling convention. An organized event assembling modeling, fashion, beauty, photography, etc., people at a convention site to offer demonstrations, lectures, contests, and other activities. It is usually sponsored by a modeling organization, magazine, cosmetics company, or school. Attendance may be limited to invitees or those in the targeted public who respond to advertisements. There is an admission fee and it can last any number of days. Also called a modeling expo or modeling fair.

modeling credit. An acknowledgement of having done print, television, film, video, or live modeling work.

modeling division. A department or section of a model-talent agency responsible for the representation of models.

modeling field. 1. the realm of activities, knowledge, and interests associated with working in the modeling industry. 2. a particular category of modeling or type of work within the modeling industry. Examples are the print, fashion show, and trade show fields.

modeling industry. The branch of business and service activities pertaining to the hiring and providing of models through model agencies for beauty, fashion, advertising, promotional, demonstrational, assistance, and theatrical modeling assignments. Also called the model industry, modeling business, model business, or model trade.

modeling market. A city, region, or country where there is a demand for a particular type of modeling or where general modeling activities occur on a regular basis.

modeling movement. A physical action or manner of moving, as a turn or gesture, by a model during the course of a modeling activity. See also *visually learned movement*.

modeling name. The name by which a model is hired and known by the industry and public. It could be the model's birth name or because of length, similarity, unusualness, or difficulty in pronunciation or spelling, a shortened or altered version of this or an entirely new name altogether. See *name change*.

modeling position. 1. a particular way of standing or posing all or various parts of the body while modeling. 2. an assigned place for modeling, as first position or last position.

modeling potential. An apparent or developable appearance and talent for becoming a successful model.

modeling school. A vocational or instructional commercial establishment where one is taught the various elements of the modeling experience. Modeling schools differ throughout the world. Some model agencies have schools structured into them. Most top agencies in the major markets have some type of model training program available to their new and inexperienced models. A modeling school can provide first experience at modeling and offer a starting point in the profession to qualified individuals at the local level.

modeling team. 1. two or more models who perform on a stage or runway at the same time. Also called a runway team, runway pair, or runway group. 2. two or more models who are associated by family relation or marriage and are referred to as a team, usually by the television or print media.

modeling trial period. The time during which a new model enters, learns, or is tested at modeling work. Also called the model training period, model testing period, or first six months.

modeling world. The realm of activities, knowledge, and interests associated with working in the modeling industry, especially as expressed in a glamorous sense.

model-photographer. Occupational title.

model-producing country. A country of the world regarded as a consistent source for new models, especially photographic beauty or fashion runway models.

model release. A contractual agreement between a model and business client or photographer stating that the right to use or sell the model's picture is surrendured for a specific or unlimited length of time for the terms agreed upon. It is signed by both parties. A parent signs in addition to or in place of a minor. Sometimes the model release is printed on the agency work voucher.

model release expiration date. The date on which the terms of a model release expire. Often this is expressed in a certain number of months beginning from the signing date of the agreement. Some model releases have no time limit and the model needs to be certain that he or she understands fully just what rights are being permanently signed over to the client or photographer. Both practices are standard.

model's account. The financial record of client billings, commission deductions, paycheck statements, yearly earnings, and the like that is maintained for each model in the accounting department of a model agency.

model's address and phone number. A model's home address, mailing address, home phone number, and possibly answering service number that a model supplies to his or her agency or places or a resume. The agency does not give out personal information to in-person or telephone callers. It does forward mail and messages as necessary. The agency may have rules and limitations regarding these practices.

model's chart. A lined-space calendar sheet or card that a booker fills in with information about upcoming bookings, go-sees, fittings, rehearsals, etc., such as time, place, duration, wardrobe, and the like.

model's fee. Payment to a model by a client for the performing of modeling services. Also called a model's rate.

model-shy. The social condition of being shy around models because of their above-average looks, seemingly glamorous lifestyles, and/or the belief that they will only date or marry the equally attractive, rich, or famous. See also *shyness*.

model's look. 1. a physical appearance characteristic or typical of a model. 2. a model's personal appearance.

model's model. A model who is a role model or career example for other models.

model's signature. Found or signed in the place provided on work vouchers, model releases, contracts, and paychecks as a necessary business procedure. In the case of a minor, the parent or guardian would sign for or in addition to the model. Whether or not a minor endorses a modeling paycheck alone would depend on the model's age and the banking program selected. A model's signature may also be found or given in the form of an autograph.

model's stance. The basic foot and body position of a model or beauty pageant contestant while standing posed in front of an audience. One foot is pointed toward the audience at a twelve o'clock position, while the other is placed close behind at a roughly two or ten o'clock position, depending on which forward foot is used. The front knee may be bent slightly toward the center line of the body and the arms, if not holding something, are held close to the sides.

model's walk. Any of various precise or fancy ways of walking while performing as a model. See also *glide, step, work a runway*.

model-trainee. A model who is going through the various stages of development and learning. Also called a student model, rookie model, young model, fledgling model, or model-to-be.

model-turned-actor. A model who decided to change his or her career to acting or to seek an additional one as an actor.

model-turned-actress. A female model who decided to change her career to acting or to seek an additional one as an actress.

model wars. Conflicts reported to occur sometimes between various agencies, individuals, etc., in the modeling industry. Media use. Also called agency wars, agency fighting, agency rivalry, contract battles, war over models, lipstick wars, high-heel wars, or beauty wars.

model-watching. The public's, business world's, and media's interest in models and how they affect the concept of beauty in society through their phyiscal appearances, the clothes they wear, and the personalities they present.

mood. An individual's emotional state or disposition toward others or events experienced.

moody look. An appearance characteristic or typical of someone in a mood of cheerlessness, sullenness, or irritability. It is predominately a male model look. Also called a sulking look, brooding look, quietly displeased look, frowning look, or lowering-one's-eyebrows look.

mother-daughter modeling team. A mother and one or more daughters who work together on a regular or occasional basis as professional models. Also called a mother-and-daughter modeling team.

mother-daughter shot. 1. a photograph in which an actual mother and daughter or two persons resembling this appear. Also called a mother-and-daughter shot. 2. a camera shot whose purpose is to produce such a phtotgraph.

motion picture modeling. Any theatrical booking in which a model is hired as an actor to portray a fashion or photographic model in a feature film or television motion picture.

mouth model. Another name for a lip model or teeth model or a combination of both.

movie commercial. A filmed advertisement for a motion picture, typically up to three minutes in length, that is played to audiences in movie theatres. A shortened version, usually twenty or thirty seconds long, is broadcast or cablecast on television. A commercial for an upcoming movie on television is even shorter and may be referred to as a network movie promo. Also called a movie ad, movie spot, film commercial, film promo, or coming attractions trailer.

movie offer. A job proposal to act in or work on a feature film or television movie.

movie theatre commercial. 1. a filmed product, service-business, or public-service advertisement that is played to an audience just before the coming attractions and feature presentation in a movie theatre. Also called a cinema commercial, advertising trailer, movie theatre ad, movie theatre spot, theatre advertising short, or theatre advertising slide. 2. an in-house commercial promoting a movie theatre or its services.

movie theatre commercial credit. A credit for having performed in, produced, or worked on a movie theatre commercial.

multiagency representation. Being represented by more than one agency, as in the case of an individual who is signed with a model agency and also with a talent agency for television and film work, or the one who is also being represented by an agency in a foreign country.

multilingual model. A model who is able to speak at least three languages with nearly equal proficiency. Two languages would be bilingual. Also called a multilanguaged model.

multiyear contract. A contract that is for a period of more than two years. A two-year contract is usually referred to as such. Also called a multiyear agreement, multiyear deal, or long-term contract.

musical ad. A radio, TV, or electronic print ad featuring music.

music video. 1. a videotaped work whose subject is the performing, especially with the use of entertaining visuals, of music. See also *video clip.* 2. such works collectively. 3. the music video industry, world, field, or profession.

music video booking. A booking to appear in a music video, usually in a silent part as a conceptual, storyline, or dance performer.

music video talent. 1. performers, other than the singers and musicians, who appear in music videos. 2. cleverness and style in performing in, producing, designing, directing, choreographing, lighting, taping, or editing music videos.

N

nail product advertising. Print, commercial, or live advertising featuring nail beauty or care products.

nail product commercial. A commercial featuring one or more nail beauty or care products. Also called a nail product spot.

name change. The changing of one's name, either legally or for professional use only, that a model, actor, singer, etc., may do because of the difficulties associated with using a birth name that is unusual, hard to pronounce, hard to spell, or identical to someone else in the same profession. For a fee, a lawyer will prepare the proper court documents for a legal name change and be present during a session with a judge when routine questions are asked and the name change application is officially signed and embossed with the seal of the court. Copies are made, which also bear the court seal, and are given to the individual as proof of a legal name change. Laws and procedures on legal name changing vary from state to state and country to country. It is generally acceptable to use an adopted name for professional modeling, acting, or other performing use without taking any legal steps, but the individual's real name, by itself or in addition to the adopted, or stage, name, must appear on all documents where legal identification is required by law. See also *modeling name*.

narration. A guiding account, story, or explanation spoken by a narrator. Also called a narrative.

narrator. An individual who provides an oral guide to a story or course of events. A narrator usually follows a planned script and does not offer spontaneous personal comments as a commentator would.

national ad. An advertisement that appears nationally, as one seen by a magazine's readers in all of its distribution markets.

national commercial. 1. a commercial broadcast or cablecast nationally on all the participating stations of a network at the same time. Also called a national spot or *network spot*. 2. any commercial that will be aired or distributed nationally, as opposed to regionally or locally.

Also called a national advertiser commercial or nationally distributed spot.

national exposure. Being seen, examined, or exhibited widely across a nation, as of a model's picture on the cover of a magazine or a personal or acting appearance on a network or syndicated television program.

natural beauty. Loveliness and attractiveness that is inborn, unaltered, and unpretending. When said of a female, it refers to being naturally beautiful or having physical beauty without cosmetic adornment; i.e., makeup.

natural look. An appearance characteristic or typical of being real, nonartificial, unchanged, unadorned, unpretentious, unstaged, or unposed.

natural movement. A modeling movement performed smoothly and unpretentiously.

natural reading. A script reading that comes across as being easy and authentic to the character being portrayed.

neck model. A model hired for an assignment requiring the photographic, video, or live modeling of the neck, usually to advertise a jewelry or perfume product in a print ad, TV commercial, or live promotion activity. Also called a parts model. See also *long neck*.

negative. A film or plate having an exposed and developed photographic image whose light areas appear as dark ones. Positive prints are made from negatives.

negotiated rate. A rate that will be determined by discussion and bargaining between the two parties involved, taking into account the specifics of the assignment. Also called a negotiated fee.

negotiation. The act of discussing and bargaining with the aim of reaching a settlement of the terms of a contract or arrangement.

network spot. A commercial that airs on network television. Also called a network program commercial, Class A spot (union designation), or *national commercial*.

new face. 1. a new face, or person, in the modeling or acting profession. 2. a new or different facial makeup appearance. 3. a new or different facial expression.

newspaper work. Modeling assignments for city or fashion newspaper advertisements or editorials.

news show modeling. Fashion or beauty modeling done on a morning, noon, afternoon, or evening news program.

new star. A new top model, actor, or celebrity.

new talent. 1. fresh, unknown, possibly untried actors, models, singers, dancers, musicians, artists, etc. Also called up & coming talent, budding talent, young talent, or newcomers. 2. one such individual. 3. a new skill or performing ability.

new wave look. An appearance characteristic or typical of a trend or movement, as in cinema or rock music, that departs from familiar or traditional concepts and experiments with or demonstrates the new. Also spelled New Wave look.

New York City apartment. Any one of the various types of apartments found in New York City (the modeling and TV commercial acting market capital of the United States) that a model or actor may occupy while pursuing a career. Examples: (All are defined elsewhere in the dictionary and apply to other cities as well. They are included as a helpful, behind-the-scenes aid for the New York-based or -bound model or actor. It should be noted, however, that New York City has an extremely low vacancy rate and inexpensive rental apartments of the type needed by young people just starting out are difficult to find. The suburbs are less expensive, but commuting is necessary. In addition to those listed, there are apartment building rental units of the one-, two-, three-, etc., bedroom type, as well as those under the protection of rent control and stabilization laws.) basement, brownstone, condo, co-op, duplex, flat, hotel, loft, men's residence, penthouse, roommate-shared, simplex, studio, sublet, suite, tenement, townhouse, triplex, walk-up, and women's residence.

New York City-based (United States). Modeling industry colleagues and activities based in New York City, a major city and seaport located at the southern tip of New York State, in the northeastern part of the United States. It is the largest city in the Western Hemisphere and is also called by its shortened name, New York. Its nickname, among others, is *the Big Apple*. New York City is the center of modeling and television commercial production in the United States and is where the highest-earning models and model-talent agencies are located. See also *Manhattan (New York City)*.

New York City suburb. Generally, a city or town within sixty minutes commuting time of New York City. Communities farther out that are linked directly to Manhattan by hourly commuter trains (up to a ninety minute ride) are often referred to as fringe, or distant, suburbs. Models and actors who commute and who want to work regularly in the New York City market are expected to have a reliable means of transportation and live in close proximity to the city. Some agencies will not represent an unestablished talent who lives too far away.

next-door-neighbor look. An appearance characteristic or typical of the average individual living in an adjacent or nearby house or apartment.

night booking. One that takes place during nighttime hours. Also called a nighttime booking or evening booking.

non-air commercial. A commercial, whether produced intentionally or designated eventually as such due to unforeseen problems, that will not be broadcast or cablecast to the public. Also called a non-air spot, in-house commercial, or demo commercial.

noncompetetive product. A product that does not compete for the same customers or market. Also called a nonrival product.

noncompetetive product ad. An ad featuring a nonrival product.

noncompetetive product commercial. A commercial featuring a nonrival product. Also called a noncompetetive product spot.

nonfashion model. 1. a model who does not work in the fashion modeling field. 2. a model who is not suited physically for working in any of the categories of the fashion modeling field. Also called a character model.

nonprofessional model. An individual who is not employed on a pay-for-service basis as a model. Also called an amateur model.

nonspeaking part. An acting role in a film, video, or stage production in which the individual is seen and not heard. Also called a silent part.

nonunion. A performer, crew member, agency, part, or production that is not a member or signatory of, or affiliated in some way, with a union or guild.

no-show. 1. a situation in which a person fails to appear for a booking, rehearsal, fitting, meeting, or other appointment. 2. the person who fails to show up. Also called a non-show.

nude ad. An advertisement in which one or more models are featured without clothing to some extent for legitimate or sensational advertising reasons. Depending on the prevailing standard, it usually does not involve full frontal nudity. Leading beauty and fashion magazines contain nude advertisements from time to time.

nude booking. An engagement to model for nude advertising or editorial photography or live for one or a class of figure artists.

nude editorial. 1. a magazine or newspaper editorial done with one or more semi- or full-nude photographs. 2. a type of nude photograph. Also called an *editorial nude*.

nude model. One who models in a state of undress. See also *figure model*.

nude modeling. Modeling done partially or totally naked, as for a photograph, drawing, painting, or sculpture.

nude photography. Field of photography in which the services of models are required for editorial, advertising, or figure modeling seminude or fully nude.

nude shot. A photograph or camera shot featuring male or female nudity. Also called a skin shot.

nudity in the dressing room. Various stages of undress that occur necessarily for male and female models in, often crowded, fashion show dressing rooms during fast-paced clothing changes and initially when makeup is first applied, in which case a smock may be available. Many times there is only one dressing room and it must be shared with any male models performing in the show. Backstage undressing is done in an atmosphere of professionalism and is a fact of life in the business of modeling. Everyone is presumedly being paid well enough to forget about modesty for a short time and just do their jobs. The most common type of nudity experienced is breast nudity for female models. A garment may require a braless look or particular bra type and changing bras to match each one would use up too much time and reveal nudity backstage while changing anyway. On studio and location shoots, a private (shielded from public view) dressing room or area is provided and may even be required, as per individual agency model booking policy.

O

obsession with physical appearance. Overly concerned, to the point of being mentally or physically unhealthy, with trying to achieve or maintain a personal physical appearance considered necessary or beneficial for one's career or personal happiness.

odd-numbered model. A model who is assigned an odd number in a fashion show production for staging or lineup purposes.

offcamera. Of or pertaining to that which is not seen by the recording lens of a camera. Also spelled off-camera or off camera.

off-hours. The time a model spends not working, as when the day is over or on weekends. Also called leisure time or spare time.

offstage. Of or pertaining to a location that is not on the visible portion of a stage. Also spelled off-stage.

off-the-rack. 1. of or pertaining to a ready-to-wear clothing item that was taken off a clothing rack, as in a department store, and purchased, as opposed to clothing that is custom made. 2. such garments collectively.

older model. A model whose physical look, either beauty or character, suggests someone of an older, more mature age. Such a model may have been in the business for a long time or started at a later age.

old-timer. A model who has been in the profession for a long (and obviously successful) time. Teen models as well as models in their thirties have been called old-timers.

oncamera. Of or pertaining to that which is seen by the recording lens of a camera. Also spelled on-camera or on camera.

one-hour fitting. A fitting session designated to be one-hour long so that an appropriate chart rate can be applied.

one-shot. 1. a photograph or camera shot featuring one subject. Also called a single shot. 2. a one-time opportunity, chance, or occurrence.

on location. On or at a chosen site for filming, taping, performing, or taking photographs. Unless specified, it is understood to mean a place other than inside or the environs of a motion picture, television, or photographic studio. Also called on site, in the field, or remote. See also *location*.

onstage. Of or pertaining to a location on the visible portion of a stage.

on-the-run repair. The hurried fixing or improving of one's personal appearance while traveling between modeling bookings.

open audition. A tryout or reading for a part in a television series, commercial, movie, video, play, or live event that is open to all who fit the requirements of the part being cast. Also called an open casting call or cattle call.

opening. 1. the beginning or first part of a performance or presentation. 2. a formal starting of operations or activities, often held as an event or celebration. 3. a job position that has recently become available; e.g., a cast opening.

open interview. A session in which anyone who believes that they may qualify can attend and be interviewed by someone in authority, as opposed to an interview that is by appointment only.

order. 1. an oral or written agreement or arrangement to purchase or supply something. 2. the item or service so ordered. 3. an oral, written, or visual authoratative instruction, command, or directive. 4. position, grouping, or organization; e.g., the order in which models will appear onstage.

original. 1. new, fresh, unique, different, or unheard of. 2. a prototype, pattern, standard, first one, initial version, or only version.

original session. The session that precedes or preceded all others.

orthodontist. A dentist specializing in the diagnosis and correction of improperly positioned teeth.

outdoor fashion show. One held outside a building.

outdoor location. A still photography, film, or video location situated outside a building or other structure. Also called an exterior location or outside location.

outdoor look. An appearance characteristic or typical of elements or activities associated with the outdoors. When said of a person, it means a healthy, energetic, exercised, possibly tanned or rugged (of males), look. It is different from a weathered look. Also called an outdoors look or outdoorsy look.

outfit. 1. a set of garments and accessories that are worn together. 2. to clothe or equip.

outgrade. To eliminate the further use of a performer from a paying production, as opposed to upgrade or downgrade.

outtake. A filmed or videotaped shot or scene, or photographic print, slide, or negative that was taken out as part of the editing process and not used in the final work. Also spelled out-take.

overexposure. 1. the excessive exposing of light to raw photographic film. 2. the state or condition of having been seen, examined, or exhibited extensively to the extent that interest has peaked and is subsiding.

overhead shot. A photograph or camera shot taken at a high-angle position looking down over or in the direction of a subject or scene.

overscale. Over the union-set minimum that is paid for performing, directing, writing, technical, service, or other-type work. Also called above scale.

oversized portfolio. A portfolio whose measurements are considerably larger than are required to display a single full-page tearsheet from a standard-size magazine on each of its insert pages. Also called a large-size portfolio, large-format portfolio, or artwork portfolio.

over-tens. Child actors and models who are over ten years old.

over-the-hill. An expression referring to someone who is considered to old to continue effectively in a job or sport.

over-the-shoulder shot. 1. a photograph in which an individual is positioned sideways with his or her face looking over one shoulder at the camera. 2. a camera shot whose purpose is to produce such a photograph. 3. a shot in which a film or video camera is positioned behind and above an actor's shoulder.

over-30 model. A model who is over thirty years old. Also called an age-30-plus model or older model.

overtime. 1. the time spent working that is not within the designated or regularly scheduled employment time. Also called golden time. 2. the payment for such work. Short for overtime payment, overtime pay, or overtime wages. Also called time-and-a-half.

P

packaging use. The utilization of a model's picture on a product's packaging for the contract terms agreed upon. Packaging may include boxes, cardboard sheets, plastic bags, wrappers, labels, decals, and stickers.

padding. 1. any soft material used to fill out or make prominent, as in a garment. It is also used to increase comfort or protection in a variety of clothing articles. 2. adding or placing material into something; e.g., padding a TV program to increase its running time or padding a script.

paparazzi. Photographers who specialize in the taking of candid and semiposed pictures of celebrities for magazines, newspapers, and other media buyers. Also referred to as free-lance photographers who follow the famous in pursuit of photo-taking opportunities. The singular in paparazzo. It is an Italian word. Also called celebrity photographers, celebrity media photographers, or celebrity photojournalists.

parade model. A professional or amateur model who appears in a parade, usually as a walking or float participant. Also called a parade walker, parade marcher, float model, or float rider.

Paris-based (France). Modeling industry colleagues and activities based in the city of Paris, the capital of France.

part. 1. an acting or performing role. 2. a piece, share, portion, segment, or cut.

parts model. A model hired for or specializing in photo, television, or live assignments requiring the modeling of one or more body parts. Parts models are hired because they have exceptionally attractive and flawless hands, legs, feet, etc., and not because they have an overall model look, even though they may already be professional models (which is how their part or parts got noticed in the first place). It is an extremely limited field with few openings. The same people work continually until they begin to show signs of aging, they move on to other interests, their rates become too high, or they suffer an injury or illness. Also called a specialty model, hand model, leg model, foot model, etc.

part-time actor. A male or female who works in the acting profession on a partial or irregular basis and relies on this employment as a secondary or equal source of income. Also called a partially employed actor or sometimes actor.

part-time actress. A female who works as an actress on a partial or irregular basis and relies on this work as a secondary or equal income source.

part-time job. Any job that a model or actor may have in order to provide extra or primary living income while pursuing a career in modeling or acting. Also called a second job or second career.

part-time model. A male or female who works in the modeling profession on a partial or irregular basis and relies on this employment as a secondary or equal source of income, as opposed to a full-time model. Also called a sometimes model.

paycheck. The weekly, semimonthly, or per-assignment payment check that is given or mailed to a model or actor by an agency or in the case of a nonrepresented job, by the client.

payday. The day of the week or month on which agency or client paychecks are given or mailed out.

pedicure. A beauty treatment consisting of cleaning, trimming, and polishing the toenails. It is done by a pedicurist.

penalty fee. A payment made or forfeited for various punitive reasons. Also called a penalty payment, penalty charge, fine, cancellation fee, or the docking of pay.

penthouse. A top floor apartment, suite, office, or studio. A building's top floor (or section) may contain one or more penthouses. It is one type of *New York City apartment*.

penthouse studio. A photographic or other-type studio located within a business space or private dwelling on the top floor or section of a commercial or residential building.

per diem. A daily payment to an individual to allow for the cost of noncovered living expenses while on a location assignment. Latin literal translation is "by the day" or "each day." Also called a per diem payment, daily allowance, or meal payment.

performer. 1. one who performs, especially in areas of physical or mental skill-based entertainment, as a singer, dancer, musician, comedian, impressionist, mentalist, story teller, reciter, magician, ice skater, juggler, acrobat, clown, or animal trainer. Also called a performing artist or entertainer. 2. an actor. 3. one who performs well in a job or profession; a doer.

perfume ad. An advertisement featuring a perfume product.

perfume commercial. A commercial that features a perfume product. Also called a perfume spot, fragrance spot, or cologne spot.

personal appearance. 1. an appearing before the public or an audience in person, as opposed to by a video- or audio-taped recording, live television hookup, or film presentation. Also called an in-person appearance. 2. an appearing on behalf of oneself and not in connection with one's work. Also called a nonprofessional appearance or informal appearance. 3. how one looks with regard to clothing, makeup, and hairstyle.

personality. 1. a person's character, manner of acting toward others, and attitude toward life in general. 2. someone having inner qualities and talents that are attractive or interesting to audiences. Also called a media personality, television personality, stage personality, or professional speaker/lecturer.

personal life. A model's, actor's, etc., life away from work. Also known as at-home life, non-work-related life, offcamera life, offscreen life, offstage life, or *social life*.

personal manager. An individual who guides and develops the career of a professional talent for an agreed-upon percentage of the earnings. A personal manager may have one or a limited number of managerial clients. A husband, wife, mother, father, boyfriend, or girlfriend may also be a personal manager. A personal manager is not an agent, but does work closely with them as well as publicists and others in the entertainment industry. Also called a career manager, talent manager, celebrity manager, agent-client intermediary, or agent-client middleperson.

personal schedule. A written or mental record of one's appointments or duties for a morning, afternoon, day, week, etc. Also called a personal calendar or personal appointment book.

personal statistics. Numerical information pertaining to an individual, as age (or age range), height, weight, chest/bust/waist/hip measurements, and garment sizes (or size ranges). Also called vital statistics.

personal wardrobe. Garments and accessories owned by a model or actor and not by the client or production company. Models usually wear clean, neat, casual clothing to go-sees and bookings and then change into the outfits that are to be modeled at the location of the assignment. A model's personal wardrobe may not contain clothes as glamorous as the ones that are modeled professionally. This may be due to financial reasons or merely a matter of having different personal tastes. Some models who are on good professional terms with designers often get to borrow outfits for special occasions; e.g., celebrity functions or television talk show appearances. The designer receives free publicity and the model gets to wear a stylish dress, gown, or other item(s). See also *interview wardrobe*.

petite. 1. short in height and small in figure. 2. a garment-size category for the woman with a smaller than average height, usually 5' 4" and under, and figure.

petite model. One who models petite-size clothing. Also called a petite-size model, short-height model, or specialty-size model.

phone messages. Business or personal telephone messages relayed to a model or actor from his or her agency, answering service, or home answering machine. See also *calling in*.

phone pocket change. The coins needed to operate a pay telephone that a model or actor keeps on hand to make routine or emergency phone calls while traveling to, in between, or at assignments. Also called phone spare change, telephone money, emergency money, or mad money.

photo agency. A business that provides stock or assignment photographs for reproduction use in magazines, books, brochures, and other printed works. Also called a stock photo agency or photo rental agency.

photo assignment. The job or task of taking or modeling for photographs that is assigned to an individual or group.

photo booking. A booking to model for or take photographs.

photo call. An appointment to appear at a specified place in order to be photographed. Also called a photo appointment, photo obligation, or photo opportunity.

photo check. 1. an examination of a photograph to determine or verify its quality or content. Also called a photo examination or photo inspection. 2. an instant picture check.

photo credit. An acknowledgement of having been the photographer, studio, rental agency, or syndicate that took or provided one or more particular photos appearing in a printed work or live exhibition. A credit may or may not actually appear on the work, as per individual contract, arrangement, policy, or chance. It may instead be a resume-listed credit. A tearsheet of the printed photo may be used by the photographer for his or her portfolio. Also called a picture credit or photo by-line.

photo exhibition. An event in which selected print photographs shot by one or more photographers are exhibited on walls or display stand panels for visitors or passers-by to look at. Examples of photo exhibition types: animal, architectural, beauty, celebrity, child, city life, fashion, flower, glamour, insect, landscape, news, nude, portrait, sports, still-life, surrealism, and underwater. Also called a photo showing, photo show, photo showcase, or photo expo.

photo feature. A prominent magazine story or report containing numerous black-and-white or color photographs.

photogenic. The quality of photographing well or attractively, as is said of a person's appearance in a photograph or on a movie screen. Some modern derivatives are videogenic, telegenic, and mediagenic.

photograph. 1. a picture produced by the process of photography and printed on photographic paper. Also called a photo, pic, print, or snapshot. 2. any picture or image produced by photography, as a transparency, negative, or hologram. 3. to record an image on photographic film or paper. Same as to lens, film, shoot, or print.

photographer. An individual who records images using a photographic camera or other device designed for this purpose.

photographer-actor. Occupational title.

photographer-actress. Occupational title.

photographer-agent. Occupational title.

photographer-author. Occupational title.

photographer-model. Occupational title.

photographer's agent. An agent or agency specializing in the representation of professional photographers. Also called a photographers' representative or photographer rep.

photographer's assistant. One of possibly several individuals who provide assistance to a photographer on an assignment. Also called an assistant photographer, photographer's helper, or photo crew member.

photographer's booking schedule. A daily, weekly, or monthly chart or page book listing the upcoming booking dates, times, locations, crews, models, clients, and the like. Also called a studio appointment book.

photographer's directions. Instructions, commands, orders, or suggestions spoken, written, or given visually to one or more models or crew members by a photographer. Examples of a photographer's directions to a photo model: "Give me a [facial/body look]," "That's it," "Hold that look," "Shake your hair," "Shake it out," "Throw your head back," "Look at me," "Look straight into the camera," "A touch of a smile," "A little more," "Good," "That's what I want to see," "Bring your chin [up/down]," "Turn a little to the [left/right]," "Move your head into the light," "Put your [arm/hand/finger/leg/foot] [wherever]," "Straight at me now," "No angles," "That's great," "Wet your lips," "Part your lips," "More," "Don't move," "Beautiful," "That's perfect," "Look over your shoulder," "Move around," "Walk [in a particular direction/manner]," "Walk and swing your arms," "One more time," "Keep repeating [a particular movement]," "Last setup," "Last roll," "Last shot," "That'll do it," "We've got it," "We're all finished," "Good job," "Good work." Also called photographer talk, photographer language, posing direction, or model direction.

photographer's fee. Payment to a photographer by a business client for the performing of photographic services. Also called a photographer's rate, photographer's percentage of budget, or page rate.

photographer's messenger. A person or company that carries messages, parcels, business and photographic materials, and conducts general or specific types of errands on behalf of a photographer. An example is a photo lab messenger.

photographer's signature. Found or signed in the place provided on work vouchers, model releases, assignment contracts, and checks as a necessary business procedure.

photographic model. A model hired for or specializing in modeling for photographs in studios and at shooting locations. Also called a photography model, photo model, or print model.

photographic studio. The indoor workplace and usually business establishment of a photographer. Also called a photography studio or photo studio.

photographic team. The group of individuals working directly on a photographic assignment, comprising ideally the photographer, assistant photographer(s), models, stylist, makeup artist, hairstylist, and possibly advertising agency or client personnel.

photography. The art, practice, or process of producing images on sensitized surfaces by the chemical action of light or other radiations.

photo lab. A commercial establishment offering the services of photographic film developing, reproducing, correcting, enlarging, and the like.

photo layout. An arrangement of photographs found in or laid out for use in a publication or other printed work.

photo session. A period of time during which a photographer, one or more models, and other personnel gather at one location to shoot photographs and engage in various related preparatory activities. For the model, these include applying makeup, readying the hair, and changing into the clothes to be modeled. Also called a shooting session, print session, still session, or sitting.

photo wall. 1. one or more walls at a model or talent agency where photographs of represented clients are displayed. Also called a client wall or cover wall. 2. a photo exhibit wall in a photographer's studio.

physical asset. A part of one's body considered beneficial because of its attractiveness or usefulness. Also called a physical attribute.

physical drawback. A part of one's body considered a disadvantage because of its unattractiveness or inefficiency. Also called a physical disadvantage, flaw, defect, or weakness.

physical requirements. Figure, facial features, height, weight, and clothing sizes associated with entering a particular field of modeling. Aspiring models should first examine the work of professional models already in the desired field by looking at magazines, fashion shows, television commercials, and the like. If there appear to be similarities with regard to beauty features (or character features for character models), age, figure, height, weight, hair, skin, teeth, and clothing sizes, the aspirant should then contact agencies representing models in those professional areas for their specific representational requirements.

pic. Short for picture and meaning a motion picture or still photograph. Also called a pix.

pictorial. Of or containing pictures.

pin. 1. any or various small, pointed metal or plastic shafts that are used to fasten items, as clothing, jewelry, or hair on a model before a fashion showing or photo session. 2. a decorative accessory that contains a pin. 3. to fasten or attach with a pin.

pinning. 1. fastening or attaching something with a pin. 2. the area that is pinned, including the pin itself.

pin-up girl. A female featured as the subject of a poster or wall calendar photo. Comes from the act of pinning up a picture of an attractive girl on a wall or door for admiring purposes. Also spelled pinup girl. A male featured as such is called a male pin-up, pin-up male, or pin-up guy. Also called a poster model or calendar model.

pivot. 1. a body movement in which one or both feet are used to turn the body sharply in a different direction. 2. to move in such a manner.

platform. An elevated, flat structure or flooring. Also called a stage.

player. 1. an individual who plays a theatrical part or role. 2. a person who plays a musical instrument. 3. a game participant.

point-of-purchase display. An advertising exhibit located in the same spot or area where a product is positioned to be picked up and purchased by consumers. It can also mean anywhere inside the store selling the product. Also called a P.O.P. display or point-of-sale display.

poise. Composure, self-confidence, ease of manner, and proper body balance. See also *camera poise*.

poitrine. French for "chest." Used as an information heading on models' composites when translating personal statistics in the English language with those in the French language.

Polaroid. 1. the trade name for Polaroid Corporation's instant-picture camera, film, and accessory photographic equipment. 2. an instant picture that was shot using a Polaroid camera.

polish. 1. refinement of style and manner. 2. perfection of appearance. 3. to refine or perfect. 4. to make glossy.

P.O.P. Abbreviation for Point-of-Purchase. Also spelled P-O-P, or p.o.p.

pop. 1. the sound or sensation associated with the sudden operation of a camera flash bulb. 2. short for pop, or popular, music.

pop-up ad. One having three-dimensional features upon opening.

portable runway. A runway designed and constructed so that it can be taken apart and moved from one location to another. Also called a movable runway. break-apart runway, or sectioned runway.

portfolio. 1. from "portable folio." Any of various flat, hand- or arm-carried cases used to hold or display papers or other flat objects. The type used in modeling is typically a zippered, handled, soft-sided case of black, brown, or neutral color, with inside storage pockets, a central ringed binder, and containing numerous clear plastic insert pages where photographs and tearsheets can be stored and displayed as a showcase of one's work. Because of its turn-the-page format, it is informally called a book. 2. a collection of a photographer's photographs, as in a magazine or picture book. 3. investment stocks and bonds owned by a person or company; i.e., an investment portfolio.

pose. 1. an attitude or arrangement of the body assumed and held while modeling for a photographer or audience. Also called a modeling position. 2. to assume a pose; i.e., to model or sit for.

posing talent. The ability to assume and maintain modeling poses proficiently. Also called posing skill, posing expertise, or posing ability.

position number. 1. a lineup or performing place number, as one, two, three, etc., that is assigned to or assumed by an individual in modeling, performing, auditioning, or interviewing situations. 2. a number assigned to a body position. Also called a pose number.

positive. A processed photographic print or transparency containing a positive image, as opposed to a negative one.

poster. A large, printed, paper sheet featuring advertising, promotional, informational, educational, or artistic subject matter.

poster booking. An engagement to model for a poster photograph or artwork.

poster model. One who poses as the subject of a photo or artwork poster. Also called a poster girl, *pin-up girl,* poster guy, poster child, or poster subject.

poster shot. 1. a photograph that will be used on a poster or as the basis for poster artwork. 2. a camera shot whose purpose is to produce such a photograph.

postproduction. One of the three work stages of a motion picture, television program, commercial, or video production. The other two are preproduction and production. Postproduction is everything that occurs to complete and ready a project for distribution and viewing after principal and secondary, or unit, filming or taping has concluded. Picture editing, sound editing, and the inclusion of any optical special effects are examples of postproduction work.

posture. The position of the body, especially of the back, shoulders, and head; e.g., a standing posture, straight posture, or slouching posture.

PR. Abbreviation for Public Relations. Also spelled P.R.

premiere. 1. the first formal public performance or showing of a fashion collection, movie, play, or other presentation. Also called an opening. 2. to perform or show for the first time.

prepping. Preparing, as for a photo session, script reading, or acting scene.

preproduction. One of the three work stages of a motion picture, television program, commercial, or video production. Preproduction is everything that occurs to develop and prepare a project for initial filming or taping. Examples of preproduction work are scriptwriting, financing, and the selecting of the director, cast, production crew, and locations.

presence modeling. Live modeling activities requiring and best served by the alluring presence of one or more attractive male or female models. The physical beauty of the model draws and holds the attention of passers-by or an audience, as at a convention exhibit or perfume handout promotion. Also called beauty presence modeling.

press agent. An owner or representing member of a business that provides representational services to clients in media and publicity matters. Also called a publicist.

press coverage. The extent to which information is gathered and reported by the news media. Also called media coverage.

press kit. A collection of publicity or public relations material held together in an envelope, folder, packet, book, box, or bag. It is given to members of the print and television media at a press conference, product showing, movie screening, or other organized event or mailing. Also called a media kit, press packet, press handout, publicity kit, or video press kit.

press release. A prepared statement distributed to the media that provides information about a product, person, place, activity, service, or event. Also called a news release, publicity release, media alert, TV alert, or video press release.

press showing. An exhibition or presentation of a designer's or manufacturer's latest collection or line of clothing, accessories, beauty products, etc., to members of the reporting media. Also called a press preview showing, press luncheon showing, press party showing, or media showing.

prestige booking. A booking, as to appear on a magazine cover, that is important because of its uniqueness, stature, influence, or the visibility it brings. Also called a prestigious booking.

prêt-à-porter collection. A ready-to-wear collection (pronounced "pret-a-por-tay").

preteen. 1. a pre-teenager. Someone twelve years old or younger. 2. a garment-size and modeling-type category. Also spelled pre-teen.

preteen model. 1. a model hired for or specializing in the modeling of preteen-size clothing. 2. a model who is under thirteen years old.

preview. 1. an advance performance, showing, or reporting, as before a formal premiere or public availability. 2. to show, see, or report in advance.

principal model. The model most prominent or essential on an assignment, as opposed to one or more secondary, or backup, models. Also called the featured model, dominent model, center of attraction, star of the shot, or star of the shoot.

principal player. A performer who plays an essential or prominent part in a motion picture, television, or stage production. Often for contract purposes, a principal player is defined as having a minimum number of lines or scenes to perform. Also called a principal performer, principal actor, or feature player.

print. 1. a positive photographic image printed from a negative. 2. anything printed with or by ink, dye, pigment, or other methods. 3. one positive copy of a motion picture film. 4. to cause to be printed. 5. a director's direction meaning that a just filmed shot or scene is acceptable (or should be saved anyway, as is sometimes the case with bloopers) and can be sent to the lab for printing; e.g., "Cut and print," "Print it," "That's a print," "Save it."

print actor. A male or female photographic model as the possessor of talent to act out various roles in front of a still camera for a photographer under his or her direction. An example is the female model who has the capability of portraying a young bride, lawyer, beach girl, corporation executive, cowgirl, store salesperson, and socialite all with equal believability for the viewer of the print photographs. Also called a photograph actor or photographic actor. See also *model as actor*.

print actress. A female print actor.

print ad. Any advertisement appearing in a printed medium, as in a magazine or newspaper.

print advertiser. The business or person doing or featured in print advertising and responsible for its cost and content.

print agent. 1. a print model's agent. 2. a print advertising agent. 3. a print promotion or print publicity agent.

print booking. An engagement to model for one or more photos that will be used in a print advertisement, magazine editorial, book, brochure, or other printed work.

print career. The knowledge and record of work and accomplishments of a model in the print modeling field.

print division. A section or department of a model-talent agency responsible for handling client photo bookings. Also called a photograph division.

print go-see. A go-see for a possible print photography booking.

print media. The various types of printed communication, as magazines, newspapers, newsletters, books, and the like. Print medium is singular.

print model. A model hired for or specializing in modeling for photographs used in printed works.

print residual. An additional payment to a model from a client for the second, third, fourth, etc., use of the same photograph of the model. If the model's services were contracted originally at a buy-out, or flat rate, there would be no residuals for additional use of the photo. The usage terms and time limit of the model release or negotiated assignment contract apply.

print work. Modeling assignments in which photographs are shot for use in one or more printed media.

private showing. A fashion, beauty product, photograph, film, video, artwork, or other-type showing that is attended by invited guests only, as opposed to one open to the general public.

procedures for submitting photos to agencies. The following guidelines are generally acceptable throughout the modeling and entertainment industries. Be certain you are submitting to the proper agency or division. For models, this can be determined by making a brief telephone call to the agency and asking what types or categories of models they represent, as fashion, beauty, full-figured, ethnic, character, demonstrator, female only, male only, children only, adults only, or children and adults. This information may also be found in the advertising pages of the telephone directory. If you have any questions about height, age, or clothing sizes, ask them then, otherwise follow the appropriate procedure given below. See *physical requirements* for ways of determining if you have a model's look and in what category or field of modeling you may be right for.

MODEL AGENCY (new models)

Mail to the proper agency or agency division four home-snapshot-size current photographs (Polaroids or regular prints): a smiling (teeth showing) full-face photo, an expressionless head profile photo, an expressionless three-quarter face photo, and a full-length (expressionless or smiling) swimsuit or similar figure-defining photo (a figure shot) in a #10 (4⅛″ × 9½″) or larger envelope with an accompanying brief, neat, one-page, typed or handwritten cover letter. Do not send oversized, overly made-up, expensively dressed, tilted head, or nude shots. Do not send slides, negatives, other transparencies, film reels, or videotapes. Professional photographs are not necessary at this point. Home indoor/outdoor photography is adequate. Do not submit to an agency requesting an evaluation fee or if its business approach seems out of the ordinary. Give your name, age, address, phone number, hair color, true eye color, and vital statistics, including clothing sizes, and politely state that you are available for an interview should the agency feel you may qualify for representation. Enclose another envelope, either the same size folded in thirds or one placed inside a slightly larger first envelope, that will hold the same photographs for return mailing to you. This second envelope should have

procedures for submitting photos to agencies cont.

the correct amount of unused postage affixed and your own address in the "send to" location. This is called a self-addressed, stamped envelope, or SASE. Mail the entire photo submission by normal first class mail. Do not send it registered, certified, or in any way that will require a time-consuming signature at the agency's end. Wait patiently for a reply, knowing that it is one of thousands of similar applicant submissions and inquiries received by top market model agencies every year and less so in smaller markets. Minors must have their parent's or legal guardian's permission to model professionally. If a minor prepares and mails in the photo submission, it would be wise to have a parent or guardian co-sign the cover letter at the bottom stating what the relation is to the applicant. This will show the agency that you are serious and would speed up the process should they want to see you in person (at your own expense, except in rare, beauty-model discovery cases). An alternative to the mail-in procedure is for the aspiring model or parent to contact the agency by phone, ask if they have a time of the day or week when they hold an open interview, and bring along the snapshots to show to the agency interviewer in person. Modeling is a profession that is based primarily on physical appearance. Whichever method is used, be prepared for the possibility, even likelihood, of rejection.

MODEL AGENCY: (established models)
Submit a professional composite or samples of work by mail or in person at an appointment or open interview. Do not mail one-of-a-kind photos or tearsheets. If applying by mail, include in a brief cover letter information on the legal status of your current agency contract or arrangement and whether you are seeking multiagency representation or an agency change. Your current agent may be able to handle both of these matters for you, depending on your situation. Include your phone number and a SASE. Do not expect your photo promotional materials returned.

TALENT AGENCY: (new and established talent)
Submit a professional, nonreturnable, unfolded, 8" × 10", glossy black-and-white, white-bordered, full-face head shot with your name (or name, agent, and union affiliations) printed on the lower front and your theatrical resume stapled or printed on the back by large-envelope mail or in person at an appointment or open interview. If seeking multiagency representation or an agency change, follow the same procedure given above for established models. Some television commercial acting markets prefer that an actor have a composite instead of a head shot. For very young children who have had no

professional acting experience, submit home snapshots similar to those of a new model. For established young children, submit a professional head shot or composite, whichever is standard in your area. Minors must have their parent's or legal guardian's consent. Enclose a brief, one-page cover letter and a #10 (4⅛" × 9½") SASE. Many agencies, even major ones, prefer not to respond unless they are interested. This is the way the system works.

producer. 1. an individual, business, or organization that plans and oversees the production of a film, video, television program, commercial, stage play, fashion show, or the like. A producer is also involved with the project's financial dealings. 2. a manufacturer.

product. Something produced, as by manufacturing, assembling, or fabricating. Product has singular or plural usage.

product advertising. Print, commercial, or live advertising featuring any type of product.

product booking. A booking to model for a product advertisement.

product conflict. An incompatibility or interference with being associated with a new or potential client's product because of the product's competetiveness, or similarity, with another client's product for which the model or TV commercial actor is currently associated with until the terms of an exclusivity work contract expire.

production. 1. the act or process of producing or manufacturing. 2. what is produced. 3. one of the three work stages in producing a theatrical film or television movie, program, commercial, or video. The other two are preproduction and postproduction. Production is everything that occurs during the actual filming or taping of the project. Collectively, it could mean all three stages.

production assistant. An individual who assists one or more administrative or technical personnel on a production.

production center. 1. a facility, complex, city, or region high in the production of film, video, music, or stage projects. 2. a facility, city, or region with a high volume of manufacturing activities.

production company. A business formed to produce one or an ongoing number of film, video, music, or live entertainment projects.

production house. A business establishment and workplace where production activities occur or are assigned from.

production staff. A group of administrative or technical production employees.

production team. A group or crew of individuals who work directly on a production.

production unit. 1. a separate, often specialized, production team that adds work necessary to the whole of a production. 2. any team assigned to work on a production. 3. a production investment share. Also called a partnership interest.

product representative. 1. an individual or business representing one or more products in advertising, public relations, distributing, or legal matters. 2. a product spokesperson in advertising, live promotion, or public relations.

professional. 1. worthy of the high standards of knowledge and skill of a profession. 2. an individual engaged in a learned or skillful occupation or activity for gain.

professional appearance. 1. a look that is businesslike, trained, correct, polished, etc. 2. an occasion of appearing before the public or an audience on a working basis for which there is pay.

professional image. How one is perceived by others in the managing of work responsibilities.

professional model. 1. an individual who is paid to perform as a model. Also called a paid model, occupational model, or career model. 2. such an individual who performs as a model in a professional manner. Also referred to as a businesslike model, trained model, or skilled model.

professional model chaser. A person who actively seeks a relationship with a particular moderate-to-high-income beauty model for reasons of financial gain or support and physical gratification. Also spelled professional model-chaser. Also called a professional chaser or one who is attracted to a model's beauty and bank account.

professional modeling. 1. modeling for which payment is received. Also called paid modeling, occupational modeling, or career modeling. 2. modeling that adheres to the normal standards of industry professionalism.

professional photograph. A photograph shot by a professional photographer, as evidenced by proper lighting, angle, focus, and composition.

professional photographer. An individual trained in photography who is paid to provide photographic services in a skillful and businesslike manner. He or she may work free-lance, operate out of a studio-based business, or be an employee of a company or organization. In major cities, a professional photographer may be represented by a photographers' agent.

profile shot. 1. a photograph of the side view of an object, especially the human face. 2. a camera shot whose purpose is to produce such a photograph.

program commercial. 1. a commercial that airs during the advertising break in a television program, as opposed to an in-store or demo commercial. 2. a network program spot.

project. 1. a planned undertaking. 2. to cast one or a series of photographic images onto a screen. 3. to speak, sing, or gesture clearly and forcefully in front of an audience; e.g., to project one's voice.

promo. 1. a filmed, videotaped, or sound-recorded promotional advertisement or announcement for upcoming programming on a television or radio station or network. Also called a promotional spot or plug. 2. a filmed advertisement promoting a current or upcoming theatrical motion picture. Also called a trailer. 3. any promotional short film or videotape. 4. short for promotional, as a promo tour or promo work. 5. one such promotional tour, job, or appearance; e.g., going on a promo or doing a promo.

promotional model. A model hired for or specializing in assignments in the promotional modeling field. Also called a promotion model or promotions model.

promotional modeling. Modeling to promote a product, service, event, activity, store, or company to others. Also called promotion modeling, promotional assistance modeling, promotional presence modeling, or public relations modeling.

prompter. 1. a person who gives offstage cues and/or lines of forgotten dialogue to onstage performers. 2. short for Teleprompter.

proof. A test, or first, photograph printed from a negative in order to examine for proof of its quality. Also called a trial photograph or test print.

proof sheet. 1. a test, or first, printing of a page, poster, or the like. Also called test sheet, trial sheet, trial impression, or galley proof. 2. a sheet photograph displaying numerous negative-size proof photographs, or frames. Also called a *contact sheet*.

prop. 1. short for property. A movable object placed on the floor, wall, table, shelf, etc., of a production set or stage. It may or may not be handled during a performance or presentation. 2. to equip a location with props. Same as to dress a set or stage.

public eye. Public watchfulness, attention, scrutiny, and examination.

public image. How one is perceived by the public. See also *clean living*.

publicist. An individual responsible for managing the public relations affairs of a client, particularly in the area of organizing and maintaining favorable publicity. Also called a publicity agent, director of publicity, public relations agent, press agent, or *print agent*.

publicity appearance. An occasion of appearing before the public or an audience in order to gain publicity for oneself, one's work, or a charity, cause, or movement. Also called a promotional appearance.

publicity campaign. An organized series of activities designed to use the power of the media to inform the public about a person, product, service, place, event, company, or store.

publicity date. An arranged outing, as to a movie premiere, with an individual who is likely to provide proper or favorable publicity for one or both of those involved. It is usually set up by the pair's publicists, mutual friends, themselves, etc. Also called a promotional date, (event) date, celebrity date, celebrity escort date, publicity outing, or promotional outing.

public relations. Field of work in which activities are performed to promote or maintain good relations between a business, organization, or individual (as a celebrity) and the public. Abbreviated as PR.

public relations agent. An owner or representing member of a business offering public relations services to clients. Also called a PR person or publicist.

public service announcement. An advertisement serving the public interest that is shown without charge on television, radio, or in movie theatres. Abbreviated as PSA. Also called a public service spot, public service message, or public service slide.

punk look. An appearance characteristic or typical of the highly unusual clothing, jewelry, makeup, hairstyles, and hair colors associated with the punk rock music movement which began in England in the late 1970s.

putting your face on. Applying various types and amounts of makeup to one's face in order to complete a desired facial appearance. An expression, or idiom. Same as making-up the face, coloring the face, or painting the face.

putting your lips on. Applying lipstick or any lip makeup to one's lips. An expression, or idiom, as in "I'll be finished as soon as I put my lips on."

Q

quarter turn. A modeling movement in which a one-quarter, or 90°, rotation to the left or right is performed while walking or in a stationary position. Also called a one-quarter turn, 90° turn, 90, or right-angle turn.

quick study. 1. an individual who can memorize script lines or action routines quickly. Also called a fast study. 2. a quick examination.

quiet look. An appearance characteristic or typical of silence, stillness, calmness, tranquility, at peace, or at rest.

"Quiet on the set." An instruction voiced by the director or an assistant just prior to the start of filming or taping activities on a production set. It is done to keep those in the vicinity from making unwanted sounds that may interfere with the recording of the performance. On large or outdoor sets, it may be spoken through a voice-amplifying device (a megaphone or bullhorn) and accompanied by a warning light, bell, or buzzer.

R

radio commercial. 1. a broadcast advertisement on radio. It may feature a model's or actor's voice and correspond to a television commercial version. Also called a radio ad, radio spot, radio promo, or radio sponsor message. 2. a commercial featuring a radio communications product.

radio commercial credit. An acknowledgement of having done voice or production work on a radio commercial.

ramp. A slanted, flat structure or flooring leading upward, downward, or around to another surface or level. A ramp may be used in conjunction with or as an access to a runway, platform, or stage. In fashion shows, the terms ramp and runway are sometimes used to mean the same thing.

ramp model. One who is employed to model clothes and accessories on a ramp or runway. Another name for a runway model.

rapid posing. Assuming planned or unplanned poses quickly, one after the other. Also called rapid-fire posing or quick posing.

rapport. An understanding, agreement, or harmony between two or more individuals or groups, or between one individual and a group. Also called chemistry.

rate. 1. a fixed or negotiated cost, charge, or payment for a service. 2. to rank or classify. 3. measure, pace, or speed.

rate of delivery. The pace or speed at which script lines are read.

ready-to-wear. Clothing articles that are manufactured in quantity in standard sizes for sale to the public, as opposed to individually made and fitted, or couture, clothing. Also called off-the-rack or prêt-à-porter.

real-people look. An appearance characteristic or typical of one or more persons normally associated with a given occupation or activity. Usually this means non-beauty model types. Plural or singular usage. Also called a real-person look, average-person look, or character look.

reception area. An open area with seating accommodations, such as may be found at a model, talent, casting, or advertising agency, where one first enters, checks in with the receptionist, and waits to be seen or met. Pre-interviews and group interviews may be conducted there. Also called a reception room or waiting area.

receptionist. A front office employee who greets and registers the arrival of visitors, answers the phone, makes appointments, gives information, etc. Also called a secretary-receptionist or receptionist-switchboard operator.

reflector. An object or device that is used to reflect light.

regional commercial. A television, radio, or movie theatre commercial that plays in a specific geographical region of a country. Also called a regional spot or regional ad.

rehearsal. A practice session before a formal or official performance, presentation, reading, or showing. Also called a run-through, walk-through, read-through, sing-through, warm-up, script session, blocking, or prepping.

rehearsal fee. An amount paid for attending and participating in a rehearsal session.

rejection. The act of rejecting or state of being rejected. It is an inherent probability of a professional career life. Those who handle rejection well go on to try again and have the chance of succeeding. (Constant rejection, however, may be an indication that you are directing your efforts toward the wrong field of work. Listen to any advice given by those doing the rejecting and other well-meaning, impartial individuals.) Also referred to as professional rejection—not personal, professional opinion—not personal, and (of models and actors) rejecting your particular look and not you.

release. 1. *model release.* 2. to give permission to leave, as from an

assignment, or to free from responsibility or obligation, as of a contract. 3. *press release.* 4. to open or make officially available for viewing, listening, or purchasing by the public a movie, video, music album, or other work. 5. what is released.
rep. Short for representative.
representation. 1. the act of representing or state of being represented. 2. a person, agency, or organization that represents another in business, legal, career, or personal matters. 3. a depiction, display, image, or portrayal.
request booking. A booking in which the services of a specific model are requested by a business client. Also called a requested-model booking.
reschedule. To change the time and/or day of an already scheduled appointment or event.
rescheduled booking. One whose date and/or time had been previously set.
reserve fund. A stored money supply that may be recorded on a model's account at a model agency. It consists of a deducted percentage from each billing. In this system, the model is paid his or her fee in the form of an advance from the agency, minus the reserve fund deduction and commission. When the client pays, the fund reverts to the model. If the client fails to pay, the fund is allowed to grow and used to pay back the advance.
reshoot. 1. to photograph, film, or videotape over again. 2. the session in which this takes place. Also called a reshooting.
residual. An additional, calculated sum of money paid to a model, actor, or other performer from a client for the re-use of a performed work in print, television, film, or radio. Also called a re-use payment.
resort wear show. A fashion show featuring warm-climate fashions. Also spelled resort-wear show or resortwear show. Also called a resort-spring show, vacation wear show, holiday wear show, or cruisewear show.
resume. A one-page, typed, outline-format summary listing a performer's name, age range, agent/phone number, personal statistics, Social Security number (U.S.), union memberships, training, skills, and performing credits. Only brief, important information is given. Pronounced "reh-zoo-may." Also spelled résumé.
retail buyer. 1. an individual who makes purchases from retail stores, catalogs, visiting salespersons, etc. Also called a retail purchaser, retail customer, consumer, or shopper. 2. short for retail merchandise *wholesale buyer.* A buyer of wholesale merchandise for a retail store,

usually in small quantities, or a chain of stores, in large quantities. Also called a retail merchandise buyer, retail stock buyer, retail store buyer, or chain store buyer.

retail modeling. Any modeling in which the services of one or more models are required for exhibiting or demonstrating a designer's or manufacturer's clothing, accessories, beauty or home products, etc., to consumers.

retail showing. An exhibition or presentation of retail fashion or beauty merchandise held in a retail store or for consumers in any location.

retail showroom. A merchandise showroom in a retail store. Items are on display or brought out from a back room and shown to consumers.

retouch. To add details or conceal imperfections on a photographic print, transparency, or negative; e.g., to spot or airbrush.

re-use. To use something over or the state of being used over. Also called re-usage, additional use, or multiple use.

re-use payment. Money paid for the re-use of something. Also called a residual.

review. 1. a print, television, or radio report evaluating the merits and/or faults of a film, video, book, fashion show, or other work. Also called a critique or evaluation. 2. to give or write or review.

revising agency card. The process of having new agency composite cards printed for a model with information and pictures that are improved, recent, or of a different style.

revising composite. The process of having new composites printed for a model or TV commercial actor with revised information and pictures.

revising portfolio. The process of removing photographs and/or tearsheets, from a portfolio, or book, and replacing them with ones that are improved, recent, or of a different style.

revolving stage. A type of stage, platform, or base, usually circular, that is constructed to spin slowly by means of a hidden motor and drive assembly. Also called a rotating stage, revolving platform, or revolving base.

role. 1. a character identity, or part, assumed and played by a performer. 2. the function or position of an individual involved in a production.

rooftop shot. A photograph or camera shot featuring or using the rooftop of a building.

roommate. An individual sharing one's room or apartment. Also called a roomie, room-sharer, apartment-sharer, apartmentmate, coresident, cohabitant, living partner, live-in, fellow abider, or fellow dweller. An example of a roommate-shared apartment is a top model agency's models' apartment. In this, which is set up by the agency, a number of agency models of the same sex share a single apartment in the city as model-roommates.

rounds. A routine course or procedure followed in going from place to place. See also *making the rounds*.

rounds list. A paper or card that lists the names and addresses of places traveled to regularly where one usually repeats an activity, for example, an interview rounds list or casting agency list.

runway. A lengthy strip of platform, stage, or floor space used by models to walk, dance, skip, jog, etc., along while displaying clothes and accessories to an audience. See also *carpeted runway, carpet runway, ramp, catwalk*.

runway model. A model hired for or specializing in the modeling of designers' and manufacturers' garments and accessories on fashion show runways. Also called a ramp model.

runway modeling. Field of modeling in which runways of varying designs are used by designers and manufacturers in the presentation by models of new clothing and accessory products to buyers, the media, and public. See also *work a runway*.

runway showing. A fashion show in which a runway is used. Also called a runway show or ramp show.

rushes. Another name for *dailies*.

rush hour. A period of time during the day when large numbers of people are walking on a city's sidewalks and cars, trucks, buses, and trains are crowded carrying more to and from work. A city's rush hour periods, usually in the morning, noontime, and late afternoon, are factors to consider when scheduling and departing to and from appointments, especially when on location.

S

SAG. Screen Actors Guild. In the United States, the union for performers working in motion pictures and television productions (including commercials) which are shot on film.

salon. A retail shop, service establishment, or store department where fashion or beauty products are sold, services performed, or instructions in their use given. When referring to a place that sells fashion products, the terms salon, boutique, and specialty shop are sometimes used to mean the same thing.

salon model. One who models in a fashion or beauty salon.

salon modeling. Any modeling done in a salon.

sample model. 1. a living model whose bodily form serves as the basis for a designer's or manufacturer's clothing and accessory samples. Also called a fitting model. 2. a hollow or solid structure or shape which serves this purpose. Also called a sample form, size model, sizing model, sizing form, or designing form. 3. a living model who is hired to hand out free samples of promotional items, as food, home or business products, perfume, or cosmetics. Also called a sample handout model, sampler, sample handout person, sample giveaway person, handout promotion assistant, or handout person.

scale. 1. the union-set minimum payment for work done, as opposed to below scale or overscale. 2. the union schedule listing graduated minimum payments for various types of performing, technical, service, etc., work. Also called a union fee scale. 3. any other pay scale, as a sliding scale or variable scale. 4. a series of relative measurements for determining or comparing sizes; e.g., small scale, large scale, or scale model. 5. a mechanical or electronic device used to determine weight.

Scandinavian model. A model based in or originally from the northern European country of Denmark, Finland, Norway, or Sweden.

scene. 1. the action, dialogue, and setting which comprises the elements of a single division of storytelling in a script. A film or video scene may be a long-playing camera shot or made up of numerous edited shots from different angles of the same script action. The terms scene and shot are sometimes used to mean the same thing. 2. a place, locale, view, picture, or display. 3. happening, focus of attention, or place to be.

scene number. A reference number assigned to each scene (or shot depending on script format) in a script. Numbers begin at one and graduate upward. Revised or added scenes or shots may be accompanied by a letter of the alphabet. The scene number also appears on the film information clapboard that is displayed in front of the running camera prior to the shooting of script action. Also called a shot number.

schoolgirl look. An appearance characteristic or typical of a young girl attending elementary or high school, particularly in the way she is dressed, how her hair is styled, and what school essentials she is carrying, as books, notebook, lunch container, shoulderbag, or the like. Other school-related looks are a college girl look, student look, prep school look, preppy look, co-ed look, and back-to-school look.

scouter. An individual who searches or maintains an observance for something. Examples are a talent scout and location scout.

screen presence. An individual's exhibited use of body movements, facial expressions, and voice in presenting an onscreen appearance and personality. Examples of screen presence types: bland, comedic, dramatic, dynamic, forceful, formidable, heroic, imposing, impressive, negative, positive, sexy, uplifting, villainous, and weak. See also *camera presence*.

screen test. A filmed or videotaped audition or interview of a performer to check his or her screen presence, performing talent, recorded voice, and role suitability. Also called a screen audition or video audition.

screenwriter. An individual who writes screenplays, treatments, stories, and outlines for theatrical or television motion pictures. Also called a movie writer, film writer, screen author, movie author, film author, or movie scriptwriter.

script. A written text in a special format that serves as the guide for the course of action, dialogue, and setting of a production. Also called a screenplay, teleplay, photoplay, or copy sheet.

script reading. The reciting from memory or reading from a paper or script-projection screen of lines from a script for rehearsing or auditioning purposes. See also *cold reading, line reading, natural reading*.

script session. A meeting attended by two or more cast members and possibly other personnel, as the director and writer(s), to rehearse individual dialogue and sometimes action of a script. It may take place sitting around a large table or on the set. Also called a script rehearsal, read-through, or run-through.

scriptwriter. An individual who writes scripts for films, videos, radio shows, play-format publications (comic books or photo soap-opera magazines), or the like. A screenwriter may also be called a scriptwriter. However, scriptwriter, the general term, does not necessarily imply writing for the screen. Also called a scripter.

seamless paper. A wide sheet of disposable background paper hung from the ceiling in a roll in a photographer's studio. To use it, a long section is pulled down and out across the floor where it is fastened, usually by tape. This creates a set without visible seams, a limbo set, for subjects to stand and move around on while being photographed, filmed, or videotaped. Seamless paper is available in different widths, lengths, and colors. Also called no-seam paper or background paper.

seamstress. A woman whose occupation is sewing. Also spelled sempstress. A male as such is called a seamster.

seasonal ad. An advertisement featuring a seasonal theme. Examples are a spring ad, winter ad, and back-to-school ad.

seasonal commercial. A limited-run TV, radio, or movie theatre commercial featuring a seasonal or holiday theme. Also called a seasonal spot, seasonal, or (holiday name) spot.

seasonal look. An appearance characteristic of a season or seasonal activity.

second tentative booking. A second booking placed tentatively on a model, this time by a different client, reserving the model's services for a particular day and time. If the first client cancels, the second aquires the option of finalizing it.

seductive look. An appearance, as of a facial expression or body pose or movement, that is characteristic or typical of one individual attempting to seduce another.

SEG. Screen Extras Guild. In the United States, a union for performers working as extras in filmed productions, including television commercials.

semipose. 1. a pose featuring only part of the body. Also called a partial pose or half pose. 2. an informal pose, as when celebrity photographers outside of a movie premiere call out to a star to stop and smile for their cameras. It is posing that happens quickly and is not held for any length of time, as would be the case under more controlled conditions. Also called a spontaneous pose or candid pose. 3. to assume a partial or half pose.

semiprofile shot. A photograph or camera shot that features a partial profile of a person or object. Also called a three-quarter face shot.

sense of humor. The capacity to appreciate life's humorous moments. Considered an advantageous quality for a model, actor, photographer, director, etc., to have.

serious look. An appearance characteristic or typical of someone who is deep in thought or unsmilingly calm or determined. It is incorporated into a variety of nonsmiling looks.

service fee. An additional payment made by a client to cover the cost of processing a business transaction. Also called a service charge or billing fee.

session. A period of time at one location during which an activity occurs.

session fee. The payment for or cost of participating in a session.

set. 1. the designated, constructed place where still photographing, filming, or videotaping occurs. 2. any designated location where a camera is set up for shooting. Also called a designated shooting area or designated performing area. 3. a television set. 4. *jet set*.

setting. 1. the time and place of events portrayed in a photograph, TV commercial, movie, play, or other fictional or nonfictional work. 2. a frame, holder, or mount for precious stones.

setup. 1. an arrangement or positioning of equipment, materials, performers, action, and/or dialogue for a planned purpose. 2. a describing of or to describe the events contained in a film or video clip before it is viewed by others, as on a television talk show. Also spelled set up or set-up.

Seventh Avenue (New York City). A major thoroughfare in the borough of Manhattan in New York City. Also called Fashion Avenue. Penn Station, Times Square, and the Garment and Theatre Districts can all be found in various areas along Seventh Avenue.

sex appeal. The quality or power of attracting the opposite sex. Also called sexual attraction.

sex symbol. An individual who is said to represent the highest or most popular standards of male or female sexuality, sex appeal, or sexiness. Also called a heartthrob or idol.

sexy look. 1. an appearance characteristic or typical of male or female sex appeal. Also called a seductive look, sensual look, sensuous look, voluptuous look, or erotic look. 2. an exciting, highly stylish look. Also called a sleek look or racy look.

sf. Abbreviation for stocking feet. Used when listing a model's height measurement (height without shoes). Also spelled s.f.

SFX. Abbreviation for Sound Effects. Also spelled sfx.

shoot. 1. to aim and press the shutter release button or trigger on a still, motion picture, or video camera recording one or a series of images. Same as to photograph, film, videotape, tape, lens, take a picture, or click one off. 2. the session in which this takes place. Short for shooting session.

shoot day. The day on which a shooting takes place.

shooting. 1. recording one or more pictures using a camera. 2. the session in which this takes place. Short for shooting session. 3. the pictures themselves.

shooting location. The place where a shooting takes place.

shooting session. An activity period during which images are recorded on still photographs, motion picture film, or videotape. Also called a shooting, shoot, photo session, still session, filming session, or video session.

short-lived career. A career that naturally or unexpectedly lasts for a short time. Modeling is a short-lived career for most primarily because of a model's eventual unsuitability for continuing to work in the traditionally youth- and beauty-oriented marketplace. This is due to natural changes in physical appearance caused by aging, as wrinkles, facial bone growth and settling, and the like. Models who age well, retaining their facial beauty and figure, have careers up to ten years and longer. See also *stepping stone*.

shot. 1. past tense of shoot. 2. one or a sequence of images, or frames, recorded using a camera. Also called a snapshot, still, shooting, footage, taping, or filming. 3. a particular camera angle, setup, or composition used in the recording of one or a series of photographic or video images. A camera shot may be brief or long playing. 4. a chance, opportunity, or attempt; e.g., a shot at the big time.

shot area. The ground and space enclosed in a shot. Also called the frame area or shot coverage.

show. 1. a presentation, exhibition, or performance. Also called a showing. 2. a theatrical film, stage production, or television or radio program; e.g., a picture show, stage show, TV show, or radio show. 3. to display, exhibit, present, or make visible.

showcase. 1. an exhibition, display, or presentation that acts as an introduction to or demonstration of one's work. 2. to exhibit, display, or present in such a manner. 3. a display case.

showing. 1. an exhibition, presentation, or performance. Also called a show. 2. displaying, exhibiting, or presenting. 3. airing, screening, playing, or running.

showroom. A room where originals or samples of salable items are on display or brought in from a different room to show to potential customers. Also called a display room, presentation room, salesroom, sample room, or front room.

showroom model. A model hired for or specializing in modeling garments, accessories, or beauty products in a designer's, manufacturer's, or retail store's showroom.

showroom modeling. Field of modeling requiring the services of full- or part-time models in wholesale or retail showrooms.

shyness. The condition, state, or characteristic of being shy. Some models and actors admit to being a little shy in their personal lives, but when modeling or acting onstage or in front of a camera they become relaxed and outgoing. For others, it is just the opposite.

Common types: people-shy, socially shy, camera-shy, publicity-shy, and *model-shy.*

sick leave. The taking of a day or more off from modeling work to recuperate from an illness. Also called an illness bookout, medical leave, medical bookout, or disability leave.

signatory. 1. an agency, producer, or production company that has signed an agreement with a union stating that it will abide by union rules and regulations with regard to the hiring and treatment of members. 2. any document signer.

sign-in sheet. A blank-space form required to be filled in by talent upon arriving at a casting session location. It requests information as performer's name, agent's name, Social Security number (U.S.), time of arrival, time of audition, whether it is the first session or a callback, etc. It is a union-required procedure. Also called an audition report form or *time sheet.*

silent part. A nonspeaking acting or performing role. Also called a nonspeaking part.

silhouette. The defining shape or outline of something, as a dress, coat, or complete outfit. Also called the outer defining lines or arrangement of outer lines.

silver card. A large reflector card that is covered or painted with a light-reflecting silver material.

simplex. A one-floor apartment, as opposed to a duplex or triplex. Also called a flat. It is one type of *New York City apartment.*

single-presenter modeling. Modeling done one at a time on a stage, runway, or in a showroom as a single presenter before a buyer or audience, as opposed to modeling in pairs or groups. Also called single-model-onstage format or alternating-model format.

single-shot. A photograph or camera shot featuring a single subject. Also called a singles shot or one-shot.

sister modeling team. Two or more sisters who work together on a regular or occasional basis as professional models.

sitting. 1. a photo session, especially one for portrait or posed-subject photography. 2. posing for an artist's portrait. 3. the correct and graceful way a model seats and unseats herself or himself during live modeling.

six-to-tens. Child actors and models who are between six-to-ten years of age.

size card. A blank-space card form found at casting sessions on which talent fills in height, weight, and clothing size information. Also called a size information card, talent size card, or talent information card.

size range. A series of clothing sizes; e.g., "dress size: 6-7-8," for a particular garment category, graduating from small to large, any of which a model can wear effectively.

skill. An ability or expertise, as in sports, dancing, musical instrument playing, or gymnastics. (A performer's resume should list only a small number of skills—enough to give a prospective employer an idea of your potential. An agent may require a more detailed list. It is not wise to have a skill listed that you are not reasonably proficient in, as this will waste time, money, and cause you embarrassment on the set.) Also called a talent or athletic ability.

skill sheet. A list of an actor's skills or talents kept by an agency in order to aid casting personnel in their selections. Also called a skill card or talent information card.

skill test. A check of a performer's resume-stated or otherwise claimed skill; e.g., ice skating ability or firearm handling. Also called a skill confirming test or skill demonstration.

skin product advertising. Print, commercial, or live advertising featuring skin beauty or care products.

skin product commercial. A commercial featuring one or more skin products. Also called a skin product spot.

slate. 1. an oncamera production information board. Also called a clapboard or marker. 2. to operate a slate board or label a shooting orally in front of a running camera. Same as to mark. 3. in a video audition, the oral stating by an actor of his or her name, agency representation, and if a child, age, in front of an active video camera just prior to auditioning. Also called an oral slate or verbal slate. 4. a schedule. 5. to schedule.

slick. 1. smooth and shiny. Same as glossy. 2. clever or skillful, as in business matters. 3. sly or cunning.

slide. A small, transparent photograph mounted in a cardboard or plastic frame. So named because it slides in and out of a projector or magnifier easily for viewing on a screen.

small-boned. Having proportionately small-sized bones in one's skeletal structure. Same as being small framed.

smile. 1. a facial expression characterized by an upward turning of the corners of the mouth and indicating pleasure, friendliness, amusement, affection, irony, or scorn. A good smile is considered an important attribute for a model to have, especially in the photographic and promotional modeling fields. 2. to show or produce a smile.

smock. A loose-fitting, lightweight overgarment worn for the protection of clothing or skin during waiting periods prior to clothing changes or during makeup applications. Also called a dressing room gown, garment protector, or makeup bib.

sneakers. A type of comfortable footwear made of canvas and having a rubber or synthetic sole. Variations are worn by models, actors, and crew members, as in a pedestrian-oriented city like New York City, during or while traveling between assignments.

social life. An individual's current status or accounting of socializing activities and/or personal relationships. Models and actors are often asked about their social lives when being questioned during print, radio, and television interviews and may find themselves mentioned in such media knowingly or unknowingly. Also called a love life, dating life, romantic life, or personal life.

socialite. A socially prominent individual. Also called a social celebrity, member of the "in" crowd, member of high society, one of the beautiful people, or blue blood.

socialite model. 1. a socialite who models in a fashion show or for a fashion or society magazine or newspaper editorial or print ad. 2. a socialite who is also a professional model. Also spelled socialite-model or model-socialite.

Social Security number. A federal government life-insurance and pension-program number that is required of all U.S. citizens (including minors) and foreigners with immigration documents who wish to work legally in the United States. A Social Security number card is obtained by filling out an application by mail or in person at the nearest Social Security regional office. Non-U.S. citizens must appear in person with their alien registration card or proper U.S. immigration form since these should not be mailed. Anyone over the age of eighteen applying for the first time must also appear in person. A full instruction sheet and application form are available free by writing, calling, or visiting any U.S. Social Security office listed in the telephone directory. The Social Security number is also used to pay and keep track of income taxes. It is also called a taxpayer identification number.

soft drink commercial. A television, radio, or movie theatre commercial featuring a nonalcoholic, usually carbonated, beverage. Also called a soft drink spot or soda commercial.

sophisticated look. 1. an appearance characteristic or typical of someone who is highly educated and experienced, worldly, or refined. Also called an intellectual look, elegant look, or high society look. 2. a complex, intricate, or highly advanced appearance.

sound check. A test for proper sound level, voice quality, or sound equipment readiness. Also called an audio check.

sound studio. A large or small room sealed from outside noises in which various types of sound can be recorded ideally. Also used for filming and videotaping. Also called a recording studio or sound stage.

speaking part. A role in a motion picture, television, or stage production in which the performer is heard and seen, except in the case of an offcamera or offstage voiceover part. Also called a speaking role or announcing part.

special effects. Unusual optical, mechanical, explosive, makeup, lighting, weather, or miniature model elements of a film, TV, or stage production. Abbreviated as SP-EFX, F-X, or SPX.

specialty agency. A model or talent agency or a division of such that represents a special category of models or performers.

specialty agent. An owner or representing member of a specialty agency or the business itself collectively.

specialty model. A model hired for assignments requiring a special talent or skill or one or more special physical features.

specialty shop. A small retail store or department in a large store specializing in one or a variety of related items.

specialty shop model. One who models in a specialty shop. Also called a shop employee model, shop salesperson model, or shop sales-assistant model.

specialty shop modeling. Modeling done in a specialty shop. Also called specialty store modeling or specialty department modeling.

speed. 1. a word called out on a film production set which means that the motors in the camera and sound recorder have reached the correct synchronous operating speed; e.g., "Speed." 2. raw film's measured sensitivity to light. 3. camera shutter speed.

spin. 1. a fast rotating movement to the left or right. Also called a whirl. 2. to move in such a manner.

spokesperson. An individual who speaks on behalf of another, a group, or a business in advertising, promotion, press, public relations, or legal matters. Also called a spokesman, spokeswoman, spokeschild, spokeskid, pitchman, pitchwoman, speechmaker, honorary chairperson, or celebrity chairperson.

spokesperson commercial. A television, radio, or movie theatre commercial that uses a spokesperson to promote, sell, or inform. Also called a spokes commercial or spokesperson spot.

spokesperson model. A model hired to act as an advertising or public relations spokesperson for a product, service, event, company, or organization. Also called a spokesmodel, superspokesmodel (media use), or good-will ambassador model.

sponsor. 1. a person, business, or organization that finances all or part of a television program, film, video, or entertainment event usually through advertising purchases. Also called a funding source or underwriter. 2. one who is responsible for another and/or who supports with money or efforts. Also called a backer, supporter, benefactor, angel, or champion. 3. to provide funding or backing as a sponsor.

sponsor representative. An individual who represents the interests of a sponsor at meetings and on production sets. The sponsor rep may be an ad agency member or direct employee of the sponsor.

spontaneous posing. Assuming one or a succession of unplanned poses for a photographer or audience. Also called ad-lib posing, freestyle posing, automatic posing, or instinct posing.

sports-figure model. A professional or nonprofessional athlete who models for a print advertisement or in a television commercial or benefit fashion show. Also called a sports-celebrity model.

sports shot. A photograph or camera shot in which the real or staged action of a sports game or ceremony is featured.

sports team. An informal weekend sports team, as in baseball, softball, football, or swimming, that is made up of agency models and possibly others.

sportswear show. An exhibition or presentation of sportswear. Also called a sportswear showing or activewear showing.

spot. 1. a short-duration broadcast, cablecast, or projected advertisement. Another name for a commercial or promo. 2. a short-duration taped or filmed information or entertainment segment on a television or radio show. 3. a position or inclusion in something; e.g., a guest spot or spot in a cast. 4. a model's or actor's designated performing mark. 5. any location. 6. a fully or somewhat rounded stain, mark, coloration, or fabric design. Also called a dot. 7. to correct or improve a photographic image by using a small brush to conceal imperfections with a tiny spot of pigment or dye. 8. a type of directional light having a narrow, focused beam. Also called a spotlight or spot lamp. 9. to place a spot on something. 10. to notice someone or something; e.g., to spot new talent.

spotting. 1. the fixing of one's eyesight and head in one position while turning the rest of the body and then quickly snapping the head at the last moment to complete the turn. A ballet movement used in various types of dancing and live modeling. Also called a spotting turn. 2. the act or process of retouching a photograph using a small brush and appropriate pigment or dye to match the surrounding area.

spread. 1. an advertisement, photo enlargement, artwork, or the like that is spread out over two facing pages of a magazine, newspaper, book, or other printed work. 2. a lengthy magazine layout or pictorial that features one photo subject or topic; e.g., an eight-page spread. 3. to extend, stretch, or open out.

spring collection. The clothing, accessories, beauty products, etc., available from a designer or manufacturer for the spring season.

spring fashion show. 1. a fashion show previewing upcoming spring fashions, usually held the fall before. 2. a fashion show held in a store or other location during the spring retail selling season.

spring forecast. A prediction or look ahead as to what the fashion trends will be in the upcoming spring season.

spring line. A variety of related garments, makeup products, etc., available from a designer or manufacturer for the spring season.

spring look. An appearance characteristic or typical of the spring clothing or weather season.

spring season. One of the four weather periods into which a year is divided and one of the two major fashion seasons. The other is the fall season. Also called the spring-summer season.

spring showing. An exhibition or presentation of a designer's or manufacturer's fashionable clothes, accessories, or other products held at a time before or during the spring season. Also called a spring show.

SS#. Abbreviation for Social Security number, which is found in the United States on various talent fill-in forms, theatrical resumes, work contracts, and records stored in agency and union files and computers. Also spelled S.S. no: or Soc. Sec. #.

stable. The represenational clients of a model or talent agency collectively. Another name for a client list. An expression.

stage. 1. an elevated structure with a flat surface used for performances, presentations, lectures, and the like. A stage is usually thought of as having a large surface area, but it can also refer to any flat, elevated structure, as a platform or runway. 2. a film or video production sound stage. Also spelled soundstage. Also called a soundproof stage or sound studio. 3. the theatrical stage as a profession, business, or industry. Also known as the footlights, the boards, or Broadway (U.S.). 4. to put on, work out, or perform. 5. phase, level, degree, or status; e.g. preproduction stage or stage in one's career.

stage fright. A sudden fear just before or during an appearance onstage in front of an audience or camera. Also called freezing, camera fright, butterflies in the stomach, backstage jitters, or cold feet.

stage left. The left side or section of a stage from the point of view of a performer facing the audience with left arm extended as an indicator.

stage modeling. Modeling done on a stage. Fashion show stages often have runways projecting out from them. Also called working a stage.

stage mother. The mother of a child model, actor, or other performer. A term sometimes used in an unfavorable sense to mean those mothers who pressure their children and make demands of and interfere unnecessarily with production personnel and processes. A male parent as such is called a stage father. Also called a stage parent.

stage parent. The mother or father of a child who works professionally in modeling, acting, singing, or any other performing profession. Sometimes used as an unfavorable description or label, as if the parent were standing in the wing of a theatre stage watching, supervising, and interfering with the performance of the child onstage. Other terms are preferable: show business parent, show biz parent, child performer's parent, child actor's parent, child model's parent, parent of a child actor/model, parent-and-personal-manager, or parent-chaperon.

stage right. The right side or section of a stage from the point of view of a performer facing the audience with right arm extended as an indicator.

stance. The position of the body and feet while standing.

stand-in. A person who physically substitutes for a star during tedious set-ups, long-angle camera shots, or (if qualified) stunt work.

star. 1. a prominent, acclaimed, celebrated, or distinguised performer or other individual. 2. the designation or title of a performer who has a leading role in a production. 3. to play a leading role or prominent part; i.e., to star or co-star. 4. anything prominent, acclaimed, or special; e.g., a star collection.

star model. A highly prominent model.

starting fee. 1. the minimum hiring rate at which a new model begins working. It is assigned by the model's agent. Also called the starting rate, new model rate, or beginner's rate. 2. the lowest hiring rate on a graduated schedule of rates for a particular type of work. Also called scale or the minimum fee.

star treatment. Special advantages, services, accommodations, or protection provided to or traditionally associated with stars. Also called star fringe benefits, star frills, star perquisites/perks, star needs, star security, or star protection.

statistics. Numerical facts, as sizes or measurements. See also *vital statistics*.

stature. 1. the height of a person or object. 2. level of accomplishment, ranking, position, status, or importance.

step. 1. a movement in which one foot is lifted and placed in a new location or position. Examples of step types: dance, fancy, fast, high, leaping, long, low, marching, matching, measured, running, short, skipping, slow, timed, turning, and walking. Also called a footstep. 2. to perform such a movement. 3. a point or level in a progression. 4. to intrude or overlap, as to step on another actor's lines. 5. any of a platform's, stages, or runway's entrance or exit steps.

stepping stone. A means by which one may accomplish something or advance to another stage, development, or position, as in professional life. Modeling is a short-lived career for most and for that reason is thought of as a stepping stone to a related, potentially longer career, as in fashion, beauty products or services, or acting. Also called a means to an end, bridge, vehicle, or springboard.

stereotype. 1. a fixed image, idea, or form; e.g., an acting stereotype. 2. to make a stereotype of.

still-life photo. A photograph featuring one or more posed, inanimate objects.

still-life photographer. A photographer hired for or specializing in shooting still-life photographs:

still photo. A single photograph featuring an image of frozen action or inaction.

still photographer. A photographer hired for or specializing in shooting single photographs, as opposed to a motion picture photographer (cinematographer).

still pose. 1. one in which the subject being photographed, painted, etc., assumes and holds a stationary position. Also called a stationary pose, frozen pose, static pose, or mannequin pose. 2. to assume and maintain such a pose.

stock photo agency. A business that keeps a large and varied supply of slides and print photographs in its files for rental purposes to magazines, book publishers, newspapers, and the like. The agency may own the work being rented or be representing the photographer and collecting a commision on the rental.

stool. Any of various types of single seats without arms or backs and attached to, usually four, legs that are found in photographic studios for subjects to sit on while being photographed.

stopping point. A location on a runway or stage where a model stops to turn, show a garment, or perform a routine or skit. Also called a stopping mark, performing mark, or performing spot.

store display. An advertising, promotional, or informational exhibit set up in a retail store.

storyboard. A collection or layout of single-page or paneled drawings or still photographs arranged in sequence with narrative information that tells the story of a proposed or completed commercial, motion picture, animation film, video, or the like. Also called a visual plan. See also *TV commercial script*.

straight copy. 1. wording that is straightforward and to the point; e.g., news copy. 2. script lines spoken without the use of voice characterization or other acting skills. Also known as straight-faced copy. 3. words, phrases, sentences, and/or numbers positioned in a straight line.

street shot. A photograph or camera shot featuring or using a city, town, or village street.

strobe light. A type of studio lamp producing brief, intermittent flashes of bright light. These can be regulated through synchronization with a camera. Also called a strobe lamp, stroboscopic lamp, or stroboscope.

student model. 1. an individual receiving vocational instruction in modeling, as an enrollee at a modeling school. 2. an elementary, high school, or college student who is also a model. Spelled student-model.

studio. A room, hall, building, or complex used for creative, instructional or commercial purposes. Also called a facility.

studio apartment. An apartment consisting typically of one large main room, a small kitchen, or kitchenette, and a bathroom. Examples of studio types: basement, brownstone, high ceilinged, high rise, loft, and walk-up. Also called an efficiency apartment. It is one type of *New York City apartment*.

studio shot. A photograph or camera shot featuring or taken inside a studio, as opposed to on location.

studio teacher. An instructor or tutor employed by a motion picture or television production company to provide schooling or training to one or more individuals. Also called a studio instructor, studio trainer, studio coach, or union-member teacher/welfare worker.

studio zone. A union-designated circular travel region, as within a major television commercial production city, outside of which, a producer according to varrying rules may have to pay an actor a travel-time fee to compensate for traveling to an assignment.

stuffing. 1. any type of soft material used to fill out or make prominent. Stuffing implies a less permanent basis than padding. 2. pushing or placing such material inside an area that will support its presence.

stylist. 1. an individual whose responsibilities may include securing,

136   stylist's fee

placing, arranging, caring for, and returning the clothes, accessories, and props used on a shooting. A stylist also makes sure that the set, models, and clothing articles look right for photographing, filming, or videotaping and makes adjustments as the session develops. 2. any other type of styling artist, designer, or consultant, as a food stylist, beauty stylist, or hair stylist.

stylist's fee. Payment to a stylist for the performing of clothing, accessory, prop, set, etc., styling services.

subject. The person, group, thing, location, activity, event, business, or idea featured prominently in, and is the basis for, a photograph, film, video, artwork, story, book, discussion, examination, or promotion. Also called a topic or main focus.

sublet. 1. an apartment leased (rented for a contractually set period of time and amount) short term (weeks/months) or long term (usually one year) from an individual who is already leasing it from the owner or the owner's rental agency. The original leasing tenant, who may be leaving on a long work assignment and does not want to be paying rent for an empty apartment, subleases it to a new tenant for that period of time, retaining the option to move back in at the end of the sublease. The subtenant pays rent to the original, or prime, tenant, who in turn pays it to the owner. New York State has specific laws covering procedures and time limits for subletting. A sublet is different from a lease assignment, which is the signing over of the remaining term of a lease to a new tenant. A sublet apartment is one type of *New York City apartment*. 2. to lease to a second party in this manner. Same as to sublease.

suite. A type of apartment, hotel room, or office consisting of a series or set of connected rooms.

summer look. An appearance characteristic or typical of the summer clothing or weather season.

super-. A prefix attached to words and meaning higher or greater in rank, status, popularity, quality, amount, or degree. It can be considered one level above the adjective top. However, the two are often used interchangeably when referring to the same person or thing. Examples: superagent, superbeauty, supercollection, supercontract, superfashion, superlook, supermodel, superphotographer, superstar, superstore, and supertalent.

supermodel. An extremely famous or accomplished model. Often used interchangeably with top model or international model. Also called a celebrity model, famous-face model, model's model, or top-top.

supermodel-actor. Occupational title. Media use.

supermodel-actress. Occupational title. Media use.
superstar. A star of the highest rank, stature, popularity, or acclaim. Also called a major star, big-name star, top-name star, show business luminary, major celebrity, heavyweight in the industry, or one of the greats.
sway. To lean or swing to one side or from side to side.
swimsuit model. A professional or amateur model who wears a swimsuit for still photo, film, video, or live modeling purposes. Also called a swimwear model, beachwear model, bathing suit model, or bikini model.
swimsuit shave. In order to achieve a suitable and acceptable advertising look on assignments requiring a female model to wear abbreviated clothing, as swimwear, lingerie, or exercisewear, it is necessary ahead of time, in addition to being a good routine to follow in the future, for the model to remove or have removed any noticeable excesses of lower abdomen, inner thigh, or pubic region body hair which may be visible to the camera and subsequently in the photographs or videotape. This is done with care using a manual razor and regular-type shaving cream. A cream remover or waxing treatment are alternative methods. Also called a bikini-line shave or bikini-line treatment.
swimsuit shot. A photograph or camera shot featuring a swimsuit, either separately or on a model. Also called a swimwear shot, bathing suit shot, or bikini shot.
swimwear show. An exhibition or presentation of swimwear. Also called a swimwear showing, swimsuit show, beachwear show, bikini show, swimwear show and contest, or bikini show and contest.
syndicated. 1. of TV shows and movies: having been sold to individual television stations for broadcast in their own markets. A TV series needs to have a minimum number of episodes for a successful syndication deal to be achieved. 2. of photos, articles, and comic strips: having been sold through a syndicate to newspapers and/or magazines for publication simultaneously.

T

T. Abbreviation for turn.
tag. A brief, visual and/or voiceover location/sales announcement added, or tagged on, to the end of a commercial.

taille. French for "waist." Used as an information heading on models' composites when translating personal statistics in the English language with those in the French language.

take. 1. a single instance or try at filming or videotaping an individual shot or entire scene. Shots and scenes may be broken down into as many takes as necessary until the director is satisfied that the best one has been recorded. A take number is assigned to each try for editing purposes. 2. the piece of film or videotape itself. 3. *outtake*. 4. to shoot a photograph; i.e., take a picture. 5. a quick look or reaction. 6. "Take five." A direction to take a five minute rest or break period. 7. take-off or takeoff. A parody or satire.

talent. 1. a special ability, aptitude, or faculty, as for modeling, acting, singing, dancing, or designing. The terms talent and skill are sometimes used to mean the same thing. 2. a talented individual. Another name for a performing artist or actor. 3. such individuals collectively.

talent agency. A representational business working on a commission basis and whose clients are actors and other talented individuals. Talent agency is a general term and implies representing individuals in any or a variety of fields of performing or creative work. Also called an entertainment agency, theatrical agency, performing artists' agency, or variety agency.

talent agent. 1. an owner or employee of a talent agency who acts as a business representative for a performer or other talented individual from a base within the entertainment industry. The agent endeavors to obtain work for the client and gets paid on a commission basis. 2. the talent agency and its operations collectively. Also called a talent business, talenting business, or supplier of talent.

talent booking. An assignment or engagement to act, sing, dance, or otherwise perform. Also called a theatrical booking, job, gig, or stint.

talent division. A section or department of a model-talent agency responsible for the representation of performing talent, usually actors. Also called a theatrical division or television division.

talent information card. 1. a blank-space card form found at audition and interview sessions on which talent is asked to fill in such information as name, phone number, Social Security number (U.S.), union memberships, personal statistics, age group, skills, and the like. Also called a talent information form, casting information card, or talent size card. 2. a blank-space information form that new representation clients fill out. Information contained on it may be entered into an agency's booking room computer. Also called an agency registration card or actor skill sheet.

talent payment company. A business hired by another to manage their production and/or residual payrolls. Also called a production payroll firm, payroll preparation service, or payroll systems company.

talent scout. An employee or verifiable associate of a talent agency, movie studio, production company, television network, music company, sports organization, or business corporation who seeks out or maintains an observance for new talent to hire, represent, or promote. Also called a talent recruiter, talent spotter, new talent director, or new talent coordinator.

talent search. One or a series of activities conducted to find new talent.

talent test. 1. a session conducted to find, select, and verify one or more talented individuals. Another name for an audition. 2. a check of a performer's resume-stated talent. Also called a talent confirming test or talent demonstration.

talk show appearance. An occasion of appearing as a guest on a television news or variety talk show in order to discuss or promote oneself, one's work, or an involvement in a charity, cause, or movement. 2. appearing on such a program to model or perform professionally. Also called a talk show booking.

tan line cover-up. The applying of a suitable colored makeup, as a *bronzer*, to the skin in order to conceal a prominent untanned area prior to photographing, videotaping, or modeling live.

tanning. Some models work at getting and keeping a light tan to their skin, as at a tanning salon, because they believe it makes their overall appearance look healthier, active, and more attractive when modeling clothes that require large amounts of skin to be exposed in front of an audience or camera. Tanning should not be overdone because of the possible long-term damaging effects to the skin. A model should consult with his or her agent before making any noticeable physical change. A new look may win or lose clients.

tape. 1. short for audiotape or videotape. 2. a cartridge, cassette, or reel of such tape. 3. to record sound and/or visuals on such tape. 4. a flexible, narrow strip of adhesive or nonadhesive material used to bind or attach objects, mark locations, attach seamless paper to the floor, etc. 5. to use adhesive or nonadhesive tape. 6. to measure the distance from a camera to a subject using a measuring tape attached to the front of the camera.

tape booking. A booking to appear in a production that will be shot on videotape for playing at a later time, as opposed to a live television booking. Also called a booking for taped television, videotape booking, or video booking.

target audience. A specific audience group at which an entertainment or advertising project or production is aimed, as opposed to a general, or mass, audience. Also called a target demographic audience or targeted buying group.

taxes. Free-lance professional models and actors are regarded as self-employed individuals and pay taxes accordingly.

teacher/welfare worker. A licensed individual required by law in some places to supervise and school children on a production set according to established regulations. Also called a studio teacher, production company guardian, or studio guardian.

tearoom modeling. A type of informal modeling done in a restaurant where tea and other refreshments are available. Also called restaurant modeling. See also *luncheon fashion show*.

tearsheet. A page or sheet torn or cut from a magazine, newspaper, catalog, brochure, book, or other printed work. It features a photograph, advertisement, story, or the like. For a model, photographer, makeup artist, hairstylist, etc., a photo tearsheet is a visible example and proof of work done in the professional marketplace. They are displayed in the plastic insert pages of a portfolio. Also spelled tear sheet. Also called a clipping, cut-out, or removed page.

teen model. 1. a model between and including the ages of thirteen and nineteen. 2. a model who, regardless of actual age, looks and works as a teen-aged model. Height and looks, not age, usually determine what category a model works in.

teeth model. One who is hired to model the teeth, usually to advertise or promote a product or service in a print ad or television commercial. Also called a cosmetic dentistry model, smile model, or parts model.

Teleprompter. The trade name for a script-roll projection device that allows a performer, newsperson, or stage speaker to read enlarged, moving copy continuously from a slanted (angled to reflect from a close-by TV monitor), transparent glass plate while appearing to be looking directly into a camera or out to an audience. A TV monitor by itself may also be used to display rolling script copy. Q-TV is a brand name and maker of such equipment.

television booking. An engagement to do modeling, acting, dancing, singing, or other-type work on television. Also called a TV booking. See also *live television booking, tape booking*.

television campaign. An ad campaign consisting of an organized airing of the same or related television commercials.

television commercial. See *TV commercial*.

television credit. An acknowledgement of having performed in or worked on any type of television production. Examples of television production-type credits: anthology series, continuing series, daytime serial (soap opera), episodic series, limited series, miniseries, movie-of-the-week, nighttime serial, news show, series episode, series pilot, situation comedy (sitcom), talk show, TV commercial, TV movie, TV special, variety show, video, and videomagazine.

television division. A section or department of a model-talent agency responsible for the representation of models and actors who work in television. Also called a talent division.

television earnings. Money earned from television employment. Also called TV income or TV wages.

television modeling. Actual fashion, beauty, spokesperson, demonstrational, or assistance modeling done on live or taped television. TV commercials, modeling new fashions on talk shows, beauty demonstrations on news shows, and game and awards show modeling are examples.

Telexing between agencies. Communicating by typed messages nationally or internationally between model or talent agencies using teletypewriters to avoid mail and live phone delays and world time differences. Telex is the trade name for a Western Union two-way teleprinter exchange service. It is one type of service available and operates over the phone lines and microwave-beam networks.

tenement apartment. A type of low-income apartment usually associated with the crowded, run-down parts of a city. It is one type of *New York City apartment*.

tentative booking. A booking in which a model's services are reserved tentatively for a particular day and time. It is made by the client as a first step in the booking process. A tentative booking is nonbinding on the client and may be canceled, rescheduled to a new tentative date, or changed to a confirmed, or final, booking. A client may have to meet an agency deadline for changing a tentative booking to a confirmed one. Different clients may place tentative bookings on the same model for the same day and time. Also called a first tentative booking, primary tentative booking, or first refusal. See also *second tentative booking*.

test. 1. to engage in the process of model or performer evaluation. 2. a single session in which this takes place; e.g., a talent test or screen test. 3. short for test shot. 4. a sound test or check.

testing. 1. the session or process by which new and established models pose without pay for photographers who are trying out new cameras and/or posing or lighting techniques in exchange for sharing in the use of the photographs for their respective portfolios. Not all photographers charge for this, but many do to recoup part or all of the cost of film, processing, and time involved. Some commercial photography studios do testings as a business. An agency will usually arrange for a new model to be tested by a photographer or studio with whom they are familiar. Also called new-model testing or an experimental shooting. 2. the session or process by which one or more actors or other performers are evaluated live or on film or tape.

test market commercial. One that is played in a selected regional area of a country first in order to test the public's reaction to a new product before making it available for sale nationally. Also called a test marketing commercial, market research commercial, or market research spot.

test shot. 1. a photograph featuring an image from a model testing session or instant picture check. 2. a camera shot whose purpose is to produce such a photograph.

theatrical agency. A representational business working on a commission basis and whose clients are actors and/or other stage performers. Also called a talent agency, actors' agency, performers' agency, or show business agency.

theatrical agent. 1. an owner or employee of a theatrical agency who represents a performer in the process of obtaining work in the entertainment industry. The terms theatrical agent and talent agent are often used interchangeably. 2. the theatrical agency and its operations collectively. Also called a theatrical agenting business or supplier of theatrical talent.

theatrical booking. An engagement to act or perform. Also called a talent booking or acting job.

theatrical division. A section or department of a multidivisioned agency responsible for the representation of theatrical performers. Also called an actor division or talent division.

theme. The principal idea, concept, or meaning of a production, exhibition, creative work, or discussion.

theme ad. An advertisement based on a particular theme, as the world of the rich, fun in the outdoors, or home for the holidays.

theme commercial. A television, radio, or movie theatre commercial using a particular theme as its basis. Also called a theme spot.

theme fashion show. A fashion show whose presentation or clothing is based on a particular theme. Examples are a romance theme show, fantasy theme show, outdoors theme show, historic theme show, gothic theme show, futuristic theme show, or movie tie-in theme show.

theme look. An appearance characteristic or typical of a particular idea, concept, vision, or experience.

thick-boned. Having proportionately large-sized bones in one's skeletal structure. Same as being large boned.

thick eyebrows. A facial characteristic, either natural or penciled in. Also called large eyebrows, big eyebrows, full eyebrows, bushy eyebrows, prominent eyebrows, or strong eyebrows.

thick hair. A physical characteristic, as opposed to having medium or fine hair. Also called thick-shafted hair, a thick head of hair, a bushy head of hair, or strong hair.

thin eyebrows. A facial characteristic that is natural, formed by plucking, or penciled in. Also called small eyebrows, fine eyebrows, narrow eyebrows, slim eyebrows, or tweezed eyebrows.

thin lips. A facial characteristic, as opposed to having medium or full lips. Also called small lips, slender lips, narrow lips, slim lips, fine lips, or unpronounced lips.

3-D model. 1. an individual who is featured in a three-dimensional photograph, stereoscopic photograph, stereo drawing, hologram, or 3-D film, videotape, or computer image. 2. any form having height, width, and depth. This includes living models, display mannequins, product prototypes, and model miniatures.

three-quarter face photo. A photograph in which three quarters of a subject's face is positioned toward the camera. Also called a three-quarter face shot or semiprofile photo.

three-quarter turn. A modeling movement in which a three-quarter rotation to the left or right is performed while walking or in a stationary position.

three-shot. A photograph or camera shot featuring three subjects. Also called a triple-shot or group shot.

time sheet. A chart on which times of arrival, lunch break, and departure are recorded on a production set so as to determine and keep track of overtime, avoid a meal penalty, and the like. Also called a time report or sign-in sheet.

title. Descriptive name or wording; e.g., a screen title.

today's face. 1. a currently popular facial look. Also called a hot face. 2. a model having such a look.

tomboy look. An appearance characteristic or typical of a young girl who currently has little or no interest in traditional feminine clothing and grooming and is rompish and noisy in a sportive way. Also called a tomboyish look.

top. An adjective meaning uppermost, highest, or finest. as in professional ranking, quality, or skill.

top model. A model who is at the top of the modeling profession in assignments, income, or recognition.
top model-actor. Occupational title. Media use.
top model-actress. Occupational title. Media use.
top-tops. Refers to those models who are at the uppermost end of the top model class; i.e., the supermodels.
townhouse. A single-family, two or more story house in a city, usually joined in a row to other such dwellings by common sidewalls. It is one type of New York City residence.
trade paper. A fashion, show business, financial, etc., industry or profession newspaper.
trade show. A promotional exhibition of products or services of an industry or profession. Also called a trade fair or expo.
trade show booking. An engagement to do modeling work at a trade show.
trade show exhibit booth. A partly enclosed area or compartment at a trade show where a company's products or service demonstrations are displayed, explained, or offered.
trade show model. A model hired for or specializing in trade show modeling assignments. Also called a trade show demonstrator, trade show exhibit model, trade show booth hostess, or convention model.
trade show modeling. Field of modeling in which the services of models are required by businesses for day-to-day or hour-to-hour demonstrational or promotional activities.
trailer. 1. a short, filmed advertisement promoting a feature film. It is shown to movie theatre or television audiences. It consists usually of selected scene segments with accompanying dialogue, music, and additional voiceover narration. The term originated in the 1920s when short entertainment and coming attraction films trailed at the end of the main feature in movie houses. Also called a movie commercial. 2. a type of location vehicle.
training. Education or instruction received, as in modeling, acting, singing, dancing, speaking, fashion designing, instrument playing, or other physical or mental skills or performing talents.
transit poster. An advertising wall or display stand poster that is found in areas of or on means of transportation. Also called a transit card, transit sheet, transit billboard, vehicle advertising panel, or vehicle advertising decal.
travel-time fee. 1. payment to a model for the time spent traveling to a booking location that is outside of a base city or other designated area. It is usually calculated at the regular full booking fee or a portion

of it. 2. payment to an actor for traveling outside of a city's studio zone.

treatment. 1. a scene-by-scene film or television story written in the present tense, describing events as they unfold. Unlike a script, camera shots and extensive dialogue exchanges are not included. Principal character's names are capitalized as they are introduced. A treatment may be up to half the length of a script and serves as the guide for its writing. Also called a film story or narrative outline. 2. *star treatment.* 3. accessorizing treatment; i.e., treating with accessories.

triple hyphenate. A person with three ongoing or achieved professions, careers, or job specialties whose occupational title, whether intended or media reported, consists of four words separated by three hyphens, as in "actor-director-writer-producer." Also spelled triple-hyphenate.

triple-shot. 1. a photograph or camera shot featuring three subjects. Also called a three-shot. 2. three photographs taken one after the other. Also called a rapid-fire shooting.

triplex. An apartment, house, or building separated into three parts. A triplex (three-floor) apartment is one type of *New York City apartment.*

tripod. A three-legged stand made of metal or wood on which a camera or other equipment is mounted.

trunk show. A fashion show production that is transported to another city for initial or re-presentation. Also called a road show, traveling show, traveling presentation, traveling exhibition, or regional showing.

turn. 1. a basic modeling movement in which the entire body or parts of it move on a circular axis or curved course. 2. to move in such a manner. 3. a responsibility or opportunity to proceed with or participate in an activity; e.g., a turn onstage or turn at modeling.

tuxedo shot. A photograph or camera shot featuring a tuxedo formal-wear outfit, either separately or on a model. Also called a tux shot or black-tie shot.

TV. Abbreviation for television. Also called telev, telly, video, small screen, tube, boob tube, box, idiot box, window to the world, or most powerful medium.

TV commercial. A filmed or videotaped advertisement, usually ten, twenty, thirty, or sixty seconds long, broadcast or cablecast on television to the public. It is designed to sell or promote a product or service or provide the public with information. Also called a television ad, commercial message, spot, or :10, :20, :30, or :60.

TV commercial actor. A male or female hired for or specializing in acting in television commercials. Also called a TV commercials actor.

TV commercial actress. A female hired for or specializing in acting in television commercials. Also called a TV commercials actress.

TV commercial agent. An agent, agency, or agency division specializing in the representation of individuals who work in any of the television commercial performing fields. Also called a TV commercials agent, TV commercial performers' agent, TV commercial actors' agent, TV commercial talent agent, or commercial agent.

TV commercial audition. A tryout or reading for an acting, announcing, singing, dancing, or other-type part in a television commercial.

TV commercial booking. An engagement to do work as a model, actor, voiceover artist, etc., in a television commercial.

TV commercial breakdown. A breakdown of a proposed television commercial production.

TV commercial career. An individual's knowledge and record of work and accomplishments in any of the television commercial performing or production fields.

TV commercial casting call. One conducted to cast the one or more parts of a planned television commercial.

TV commercial casting photography. The shooting of composite and resume photographs of television commercial talent.

TV commercial center. A facility, city, or region high in the production of television commercials.

TV commercial children. Children who appear or are heard in television commercials. Also called TV commercial kids or TV advertising children.

TV commercial contract. 1. a contract to perform in, produce, or do production work on a television commercial. 2. a contract or contract clause between an agent and talent stating that the agent will represent talent in obtaining work in television commercials.

TV commercial copy. 1. wording for a television commercial that is to be spoken or superimposed on the screen. 2. a film or videotape duplicate of a television commercial.

TV commercial credit. A credit for having performed in, produced, or worked on a television commercial production.

TV commercial director. A film or video director hired for or specializing in directing the filming or taping of television commercials. Also called a TV commercials director or TV specialty director.

TV commercial foreign-use fee. A fee paid by a client to an actor or model when a commercial is designated for airing in a foreign country.

TV commercial interview. A meeting between one or more production or casting personnel and talent to discuss a possible performing assignment in a television commercial.

TV commercial look. 1. an appearance suitable or ideal for appearing in one or more television commercials. 2. an appearance characteristic or typical of the traditional television commercial format; i.e., having the look of a TV commercial or obviously being a TV commercial.

TV commercial model. A model who performs as a beauty, fashion, or spokesperson model in television commercials. Also called a TV commercial model-actor, TV commercial model-actress, commercial model, or TV spokesmodel.

TV commercial modeling. Advertising acting done in a television commercial as a beauty, fashion, or spokes model displaying or speaking about clothing, makeup, perfume, shampoo, hair coloring, or the like. Also called TV commercial beauty modeling or TV spokesmodeling.

TV commercial payment receipt. A document listing payment and usage information that accompanies a television commercial talent's paycheck.

TV commercial potential. 1. an apparent or developable ability for doing performing or voiceover work in television commercials. 2. a TV commercial's selling power.

TV commercial producer. A film or video producer hired for or specializing in organizing and supervising the cost and production of television commercials. Also called a TV commercials producer.

TV commercial rate. 1. the fee for television commercial acting, voiceover, or production work. Also called a TV commercial scale payment. 2. the fee charged for airing a television commercial.

TV commercial residual. A residual paid for the additional airing of acting or voiceover work done in a television commercial. Also called a commercial re-use payment.

TV commercial script. One or more sheets of paper or cue card with dialogue and sometimes action for a television commercial typed or hand printed on it. A storyboard is also considered part of or a complete television commercial script.

TV commercial session. 1. an occasion of filming, videotaping, or audiotaping a television commercial. Also called a TV commercial shoot. 2. a session in which talent is auditioned or interviewed for a possible television commercial acting or voiceover job.

TV commercial talent. 1. the actors, announcers, singers, dancers, and animals who appear or are heard in television commercials. 2.

one such individual or animal. 3. the ability to act or perform well in television commercials.

TV commercial title. 1. the story or reference name assigned to a television commercial. 2. a word, phrase, sentence, number, or logo, as a product name, sale phrase, or price that appears onscreen during a television commercial. Also called a commercial screen caption, commercial screen copy, or commercial screen graphics.

TV commercial type. 1. of a kind suitable for television commercial performing work. 2. a particular kind of television commercial.

TV commercial wardrobe allowance. A payment to an actor when personal clothing is worn in front of the camera on a television commercial shooting. The amount of payment depends on what type of clothing is involved, as evening or nonevening wear. Also called a TV commercial wardrobe compensation.

TV commercial wardrobe call. A wardrobe call for a television commercial oncamera performing job.

TV go-see. The appointment or act of going to see someone who is auditioning or interviewing talent for television work.

two-shot. A photograph or camera shot featuring two subjects. Also called a doubles shot.

typecast. To cast or have been cast as an actor once or continually according to a particular physical or image type rather than the ability to assume different performing roles.

type classification. The role playing or physical-feature category designation of a model or actor.

type conflict. 1. a situation arising when an actor's looks, voice, or performing style clashes with one or more other actors or the character type being portrayed. This may be intentional or unintentional. 2. a situation resulting from an agency's representation of a number of actors of the same extreme character type who compete against each other continually for the same roles. Also called a representation conflict.

U

UDA. Union Des Artists. In Canada, a union for performers working in the French-speaking market.

ugly-up. To make oneself less attractive by removing or adding makeup or lowering one's standard of clothing or hairstyle for a short time. An example is putting on a disguise so as not to be recognized by fans and celebrity photographers in public. Same as to unbeautify or unglamorize.

umbrella reflector. A type of collapsable reflector resembling and operating like an outdoor rain umbrella. It is mounted on an adjustable pole stand and has an attached lamp that is shone continually or flashed, bouncing light onto a set or photographic subject.

under-sixes. Child actors and models who are under six years old.

understudy. A rehearsed, substitute performer.

underwear ad. An advertisement featuring one or more underwear products. Also called an undergarment ad, underclothing ad, or lingerie ad.

underwear model. A model hired for an assignment requiring the modeling of one or more underwear products, as for a magazine or newspaper ad, store display card, catalog picture, or in a live fashion showing. Also called an undergarment model, underclothing model, or lingerie model.

underwear modeling. Field of modeling in which the services of models are required by manufacturers and designers for the modeling of underwear products.

union. An organization representing workers in a particular occupation in wage, benefit, and working-condition contracts and also in employee-management disputes. Also called a labor organization, guild, federation, league, society, alliance, brotherhood, or professional association.

union card. A printed membership card issued to members of a union. It contains, among other information, the member's name and identification number. Also called a guild card.

union dues. Payments made at regular intervals to a union by each of its card-carrying members in order to fund the union's operation and various membership programs. The word dues has singular or plural usage.

union fee scale. A schedule of graduated minimum payments for work assignments done within a union's juristiction. Also called a union rate scale, union pay scale, union sliding scale, or theatrical compensation scale.

union initiation fee. A one-time payment to a union, usually in the hundreds of dollars (U.S.), required to be made by a new member when first joining.

union member. An individual who is officially in the ranks of union membership. See also *guild member, signatory*.

union membership computer. A computer system used by a union to store and retrieve necessary information about its members, including current agency representation or answering service phone number. Also called a membership information computer or membership records computer.

union representative. An employee of a union who represents the interests of its membership. Also called a union official, union spokesperson, or union contract negotiator.

union rule book. A printed book or booklet detailing union rules. Also called a union handbook.

unit. 1. a film or tape crew or team. Also called a company. 2. one of a number of things, products, or people; e.g., a TV audience population unit or apartment unit. 3. an investment share in a project or production.

unposed look. An appearance characteristic or typical of a natural, unstaged body position. Also called an unstaged look, unpretentious look, or natural look.

unprofessional model. An untrained, careless, or unbusinesslike model.

upgrade. To raise the status of a performer in a production to a greater role and/or pay level.

upstage. 1. at or toward the back of a stage, runway, or platform. 2. to divert attention or outdo.

upstage foot. The foot positioned closest to or moving toward the back of a stage initially.

usage. How something is used, as a model's photographic image by a client.

V

vacation leave. The taking of a day or more off from modeling work to go on a vacation. Also called a vacation bookout.

video. 1. an entertainment, educational, informational, or promotional work produced originally on or transferred subsequently to videotape. 2. such works collectively. 3. the video industry, world, field, or profession. Also called videodom. 4. TV pictures, visuals, or graphics.

video actor. A male or female who acts in videos. Also called a video performer.

video actress. A female who acts in videos.

video artists' model. An individual who models in person or by way of photographs for artists whose creative medium is video. Also called a video artist's model, video artist's subject, video art model, or video model.

video-assisted fashion show. A fashion show production that uses one or more television sets or large-screen TVs in the background or on the sides with accompanying recorded or live television images shown on them to add excitement, creativeness, and/or symbolism to the presentation.

video audition. An audition in which performers are recorded individually or collectively on videotape for later viewing during the casting decision-making process. A video audition is done to check an individual's television screen presence, performing talent, voice on tape, and role suitability. Because it is less expensive and faster, it may be done in place of a filmed screen test. Also called a video screen test, video test, or taped audition.

video booking. An engagement to model, act, dance, exercise, or do other-type work in a video production. See also *videotape booking*.

video camera. 1. an attached, handheld, or shoulder-mounted camera that uses electronic and motor-driven elements to record both visual and audio on a videotape cartridge or cassette inserted into it or a connected unit. 2. any television camera.

video clip. 1. a portion of a videotaped work. 2. another name for a music video. Also called a music video clip, music clip, video album clip, or video album cut.

videographer. One who records or creates single or moving images on videotape for the medium of television using a camera and/or computer system designed for this purpose.

video promo. A videotaped work of short duration that promotes something.

video session. One in which videotape is used as the primary recording medium. Also called a tape session, taping session, or video shoot.

videotape. 1. a flexible plastic tape coated with an iron-oxide substance.

It is designed for recording and playing back color and black-and-white images and sound through magnetic reorganization and reading of the coating's sensitive particles. Also spelled video tape. 2. to record images with or without accompanying sound on such tape. 3. a videocassette.

videotape booking. An engagement to perform in or work on an entertainment, educational, informational, or promotional videotape production as a model, actor, dancer, narrator, or in some other capacity. See also *tape booking*.

visually learned movement. A modeling movement that is learned by observing an experienced individual perform it first and then imitating that action. See also *mirror practice*.

visual sell. The advertising or promoting of a product in such a way as to make one or more of the product's visual features, as the bubbling of soda, steaming of soup, ripe color of fruit, design of a car, or style and fit of jeans highly prominent and appealing to viewers.

vital statistics. Important basic numerical information about an individual, as body weight and measurements and clothing sizes. See also *personal statistics*.

VO. Abbreviation for Voiceover. Also spelled V.O. or v.o.

voice cue. A word, phrase, or vocal sound that acts as a cue. Also called a verbal cue or voice signal.

voiceover. Narration, commentary, dialogue, or vocal sounds that are spoken or sung over the visual events and/or natural background sounds of a filmed, videotaped, audiotaped, or live activity. Also spelled voice-over.

voiceover artist. An individual, normally unseen when performing, hired for or specializing in doing voiceover work. Also called a voice actor, *announcer*, offscreen narrator, or (as a vocalist) commercial background singer.

voiceover division. A section or department of a talent or theatrical agency responsible for the representation of voiceover artists. Also called a commercial voiceover division.

voiceover talent. 1. an individual who does voiceovers or such individuals collectively. 2. a special ability or aptitude for performing voiceovers, as a distinctive announcing voice, attention-grabbing voice, serious announcing voice, comedic announcing voice, imitative voice, or cartoon character voice.

voice/speech lessons. Private or group instructions in voice projection, quality, and clarity; speech articulation; accent losing; accent learning; voice characterization; voice imitation; announcing; and singing that an actor or actor-model takes necessarily in order to prepare for a part or to further enhance or expand his or her career.

voice test. A test to determine quality, suitability, or sound level of a performer's recorded, amplified, or live voice before or during a performance or audition.

voucher. An agency-originated, multicopy, fill-in receipt form that is carried by a model and used to document booking arrival and departure times, rate, amount owed by the client, any overtime, date, location of assignment, if it is a fitting or rehearsal, model's name, client's name and address, client contact or department, model agency's address and phone number, model's signature, client's signature, and possibly model release. The model fills in as much of the required pre-information as possible or is standard in the blank spaces on the form. In the case of a child model, the parent does it. The pre-information for the voucher is obtained by the model from his or her agency, usually over the telephone. At the end of the booking, the client and model sign in the appropriate spaces and the client receives a copy. A parent may be required to sign in addition to or in place of a minor-aged model. The model keeps one copy and mails or hands in the agency's copy, which is then used in preparing the client billing. Also called a work voucher.

voucher book. A book containing a supply of removable vouchers. Each represented model of an agency receives at least one. An additional supply may be provided or available for picking up at the agency. Also called a voucher/model release book or voucher pad.

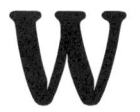

W

waiting room. A room where one waits before performing or being met, interviewed, or auditioned.

wakeup call. A prearranged, usually early morning, telephone call that wakes up a model or actor on the day of a very important booking or travel appointment.

walk-on. 1. a small, nonspeaking acting part in which the performer walks onstage or on the set as the script indicates during the course of a production. Also called a silent bit part. 2. the performer playing this role. Also called an extra or silent bit player.

walk-up. 1. a type of apartment situated above ground level in a building with no elevator and requiring a walk up one or more flights of stairs to reach it. Also spelled walkup. It is one type of *New York City apartment*. 2. the building containing this and similar apartments.

wardrobe. A collection or supply of clothes, costumes, and/or accessories. See also *personal wardrobe*.

wardrobe allowance. An additional payment to an actor to compensate for wearing personal clothes on a job. See also *TV commercial wardrobe allowance*.

wardrobe assistant. An individual who assists in the handling and caring of the wardrobe used on a production.

wardrobe call. A request or notice to an individual to arrive at a particular time and place for a theatrical or fashion fitting. Also called a costume call or wardrobing appointment.

wardrobe department. A section of a film or tape production house, studio, or performing stage theatre responsible for storing, caring for, and/or creating different types of production wardrobes.

warning light. 1. a revolving, flashing, or steady bright light that warns of current or impending filming, videotaping, audiotaping, or broadcasting. Also called a stand-by light, filming-in-progress light, taping-in-progress light, or on-the-air light. 2. a damage or trouble-indicating light. 3. a glowing light on a camera that indicates the unit is operating. Also called a camera cue light or power-on light. 4. a glowing light on an electronic flash that indicates the unit is charging or charged. Also called a flash charging light or flash ready light.

weather-permitting booking. A booking, as for an outdoor modeling assignment, that will take place only if the weather on that day and time is not hindered by rain, snow, high winds, or intolerably cold temperature. Both parties (the agency and client or model and client in the case of a nonrepresented model) contact each other by phone to make the final determination. If the booking is canceled, an *alternate booking*, if it was not made beforehand, is arranged. There may be a penalty fee, especially if the top markets, for canceling a weather-permitting booking, since the model could have been booked by another client for indoor work on that same day and time, and because a booking is a type of contract, whether oral or in writing. Also called a weather-permit booking, weather permit, w.p. booking, or *WP*.

weather-permitting cancellation fee. A cancellation fee, usually a portion of the model's full rate, required to be paid by a client for canceling a confirmed weather-permitting booking after an agreed upon time limit, or deadline, for canceling or rescheduling has expired. Also called a w.p. booking cancellation fee.

weight chart. See *height-weight chart*.

wetting down. Spraying, sprinkling, sponging, rubbing, or otherwise placing water, oil, or other liquid on the skin or hair of a model or actor before photographing or taping to create any of a variety of wet looks, as sweating from physical exercise or wetness from a rainstorm, bathroom shower, or crying.

"Wet your lips." A spoken instruction from a photographer requesting a female model to moisten her lips using the natural saliva in her mouth in order to give them an undried, glossy look and therefore a highlighted one as well. Also said: "Moisten your lips," "Lick your lips," "Add a shine to your lips," "Do this/Go like this [photographer demonstrates]."

whirl. 1. a quick spin to the left or right. Also called a whirlabout. 2. to move in such a manner; e.g., holding the edge of a garment out and whirling.

wholesale buyer. An individual responsible for analyzing market trends and then purchasing designers' and manufacturers' clothing or nonclothing products directly or from a distributor at wholesale prices for sale at one or through a chain of department stores, clothing stores, specialty shops, a catalog house, or the like. Also called a quantity purchaser. See also *retail buyer*.

wholesale fashion house. A fashion house dealing in the design, production, and/or selling of wholesale fashion. Also called a fashion wholesaler, fashion distributor, fashion jobber, or fashion contractor.

wholesale modeling. Any modeling of a designer's or manufacturer's products for one or more wholesale buyers.

wholesale showing. An exhibition or presentation of a designer's or manufacturer's clothing, accessories, or other products to one or more wholesale buyers.

wholesale showroom. A room used for the display or presentation of wholesale merchandise.

wholesome look. An appearance characteristic or typical of being physically, mentally, and morally healthy and beneficial; fit in mind and body; sound, good, clean and fresh; fresh and natural; or attractively fresh.

wide-set eyes. A physical characteristic associated with female facial beauty. Successful photo models tend to have average-to-wide-set eyes.

wild look. An appearance characteristic or typical of being untamed, unrestrained, unrestricted, rebellious, outrageous, messed up, or ruffled up.

wild spot. A television commercial advertising a national product that is shown wildly across the country in different markets by individual network-affiliated or independent stations at different times selected and paid for by the advertiser. The actual playing of the spot is done at the local station and is not part of, although may be inserted into for local audiences, the programming and commercials fed to the station by the national network, if the station is an affiliate. Also spelled wildspot. Also called a locally aired national product commercial.

wild spot payment scale. A union pay scale for determining payment to television commercial actors who appear in wild spots.

windblown look. An appearance characteristic or typical of being blown about or to one side freely or wildly by the wind. Also spelled windblown look. Also called a windswept look.

wind machine. A large fan placed just off the set and used to create the effect of wind in a scene.

wing it. To improvise or do something without having rehearsed.

wings. The two sections of a theatre stage to the far left and right.

winter look. An appearance characteristic or typical of the winter clothing or weather season.

woman-child. 1. a descriptive phrase referring to a young adult female who possesses a combination of womanly features and childlike qualities. 2. a womanly child. See also *child-woman*.

women's division. A section or department of a model agency responsible for the representation of women. Also called a women's section, women's department, or female division.

women's residence. A type of apartment or rooming house run usually by a religious or civic organization and offering low-priced, protected living accommodations for women only within a large city. Some basic facilities have to be shared and there are in-house rules to follow. Rooms may have to be reserved in advance by requesting and filling out an application. A good city guidebook should list specific organizations, locations, and length-of-stay information. Also called a women's hotel. A room in a women's residence is one type of *New York City apartment*.

work a runway. To put conscious effort into the use of body movements, turns, and the like while walking, dancing, etc., up and down a runway modeling an outfit to an audience. An expression.

working weight. The personal weight level at which one looks and works best, as opposed to a vacation weight or maternity weight. Also called a modeling weight or ideal performing weight.

work permit. 1. an official document issued by a government agency that allows a minor to work in modeling, TV commercials, films, videos, and the like, and under certain conditions. Not required everywhere. Also called a child's working papers. 2. an official document that permits and regulates the employment of a foreigner in the country that issued it. A tax is usually deducted from income received. Also called a foreign work permit or foreign working papers.

work vacation. A location assignment, as in a distant or foreign city or at a tourist resort, that doubles as a vacation for those involved. Also called a working vacation.

WP. Abbreviation for Weather Permitting or Weather Permit. Also spelled W.P., wp, or w.p.

wrap. 1. a director's direction meaning to finish, conclude, or complete an activity; e.g., "Wrap it up." 2. the state or condition of being finished, concluded, or completed; e.g., "That's a wrap," "It's a wrap." 3. an article of outer clothing.

writing appointment. A private fashion showing scheduled to allow one or a group of buyers the opportunity to examine merchandise more closely and write up orders.

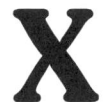

X

X-rated. 1. a rating issued by a country's or entertainment industry's film review board specifying or suggesting that individuals under a certain age are not or should not be permitted to view a particular theatrical film because of its extremely violent and/or explicitly sexual content. Age limits for the X-rating vary from country to country and may be raised by local governments to be more in line with their own community standards. 2. of, like, or pertaining to X-rated material, specifically, anything of a sexually explicit nature, as videos, magazines, dialogue, etc. Also called adult-oriented or for adults only.

Y

yeux. French for "eyes." Used as an information heading on models' composites when translating personal facts (eye color) in the English language with those in the French language.

"You look different than your pictures." The saying and situation female models and actors who wear disguising amounts of makeup on the job face when they remove it in between bookings or after work and go out in public wearing none or less and are recognized. Also, photographs and screen images are flat and two dimensional, as opposed to three-dimensional real life. Other sayings experienced are "You don't look like your pictures," "You look different in real life," "You look familiar," "Are you a model?," "Are you that actor . . . ?," "Is your name . . . ?"

young actor. 1. a male or female who has yet to become fully established in the profession of acting. 2. an actor who is of a young age. Also called a child actor. 3. an actor with young looks. Also called a young-looking actor or youthful actor.

young actress. 1. a female who has yet to become fully established in the profession of acting. 2. a child actress. 3. a young-looking actress.

young model. 1. a male or female who has yet to become fully established in the profession of modeling. Also called a new model, newcomer, beginning model, fledgling model, up & coming model, rookie model, model-trainee, or student model. 2. a model who is of a young age. Also called a child model. 3. a model with young looks. Also called a young-looking model or youthful model.

young photographer. 1. a male or female who has yet to become fully established in the profession of photography. Also called a new photographer, beginning photographer, rookie photographer, or novice photographer. 2. a photographer who is of a young age.

Z

Zed card. Another name for the composite card, after its originator, a Mr. Zed from Germany. Also spelled Zed Card or ZED card.

zoom shot. 1. a film or video camera shot using a zoom lens. In it, magnification of the subject can be varied by control of the lens to bring the subject in close or far away while still staying in focus and the camera remaining stationary. 2. a film or video camera shot in which the camera physically moves toward or away from the subject, as by the use of a dolly or track.

7199